Modern Approaches in Cardiovascular Disease Therapeutics: From Molecular Genetics to Tissue Engineering

Modern Approaches in Cardiovascular Disease Therapeutics: From Molecular Genetics to Tissue Engineering

Editors

Panagiotis Mallis
Efstathios Michalopoulos

MDPI • Basel • Beijing • Wuhan • Barcelona • Belgrade • Manchester • Tokyo • Cluj • Tianjin

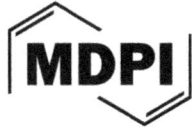

Editors
Panagiotis Mallis
Research Foundation Academy of Athens (BRFAA)
Greece

Efstathios Michalopoulos
Biomedical Research Foundation Academy of Athens (BRFAA)
Greece

Editorial Office
MDPI
St. Alban-Anlage 66
4052 Basel, Switzerland

This is a reprint of articles from the Special Issue published online in the open access journal *Bioengineering* (ISSN 2306-5354) (available at: https://www.mdpi.com/journal/bioengineering/special_issues/cardiovascular_disease_therapeutics).

For citation purposes, cite each article independently as indicated on the article page online and as indicated below:

LastName, A.A.; LastName, B.B.; LastName, C.C. Article Title. *Journal Name* **Year**, *Volume Number*, Page Range.

ISBN 978-3-0365-2436-8 (Hbk)
ISBN 978-3-0365-2437-5 (PDF)

Cover image courtesy of Panagiotis Mallis

© 2021 by the authors. Articles in this book are Open Access and distributed under the Creative Commons Attribution (CC BY) license, which allows users to download, copy and build upon published articles, as long as the author and publisher are properly credited, which ensures maximum dissemination and a wider impact of our publications.

The book as a whole is distributed by MDPI under the terms and conditions of the Creative Commons license CC BY-NC-ND.

Contents

About the Editors . . . . **vii**

Preface to "Modern Approaches in Cardiovascular Disease Therapeutics: From Molecular Genetics to Tissue Engineering" . . . . **ix**

Panagiotis Mallis, Efstathios Michalopoulos and Catherine Stavropoulos-Giokas
Modern Approaches in Cardiovascular Disease Therapeutics: From Molecular Genetics to Tissue Engineering
Reprinted from: *Bioengineering* **2021**, *8*, 174, doi:10.3390/bioengineering8110174 . . . . **1**

Panagiotis Mallis, Dimitrios P. Sokolis, Michalis Katsimpoulas, Alkiviadis Kostakis, Catherine Stavropoulos-Giokas and Efstathios Michalopoulos
Improved Repopulation Efficacy of Decellularized Small Diameter Vascular Grafts Utilizing the Cord Blood Platelet Lysate
Reprinted from: *Bioengineering* **2021**, *8*, 118, doi:10.3390/bioengineering8090118 . . . . **5**

Anna Garcia-Sabaté, Walaa Kamal E. Mohamed, Jiranuwat Sapudom, Aseel Alatoom, Layla Al Safadi and Jeremy C. M. Teo
Biomimetic 3D Models for Investigating the Role of Monocytes and Macrophages in Atherosclerosis
Reprinted from: *Bioengineering* **2020**, *7*, 113, doi:10.3390/bioengineering7030113 . . . . **27**

Foteini K. Kozaniti, Despoina Nektaria Metsiou, Aikaterini E. Manara, George Athanassiou and Despina D. Deligianni
Recent Advancements in 3D Printing and Bioprinting Methods for Cardiovascular Tissue Engineering
Reprinted from: *Bioengineering* **2021**, *8*, 133, doi:0.3390/bioengineering8100133 . . . . **47**

Panagiotis Mallis, Alkiviadis Kostakis, Catherine Stavropoulos-Giokas and Efstathios Michalopoulos
Future Perspectives in Small-Diameter Vascular Graft Engineering
Reprinted from: *Bioengineering* **2020**, *7*, 160, doi:10.3390/bioengineering7040160 . . . . **61**

About the Editors

Panagiotis Mallis, MSc, PhD, is serving as an Associate Scientist of the Hellenic Cord Blood Bank of the Biomedical Research Foundation Academy of Athens, Greece. His master diploma and PhD were focused in the field of the Small-Diameter Vascular Graft Engineering. Since 2012, he has been a member of the Hellenic Cord Blood Bank, and his research interests involve the development of vascular grafts using state-of-the-art tissue engineering methods, investigating the immunobiology of stem cells, including hematopoietic stem cells (HSCs) and mesenchymal stromal cells (MSCs). In recent years, he has focused on the publication of scientific articles, participated in conferences and presented invited talks. To date, he has published more than 25 articles (original research, review articles, editorials, etc.). He has participated as first author in more than 15 articles that are available in PubMed (MEDLINE). Additionally, he has carried out several peer-reviews for a great number of international journals. Currently, he is serving as Guest Editor and member of the Topical Advisory Panel of the Bioengineering (Basel). Last year, he published the Special Issue "Stem Cell and Biological Scaffold Engineering" (printed version).

Efstathios Michalopoulos, MSc, PhD, is serving as the quality manager of the Hellenic Cord Blood Bank of the Biomedical Research Foundation Academy of Athens, Greece. He uses his training and experience in biomedical engineering and researches, alongside his colleagues, the expansion of hematopoietic stem cells from cord blood, the ability of angiogenesis of human umbilical cord blood cells in a three-dimensional environment and the regenerative role of adipose stem cells and bone marrow in animal models. Additionally, he has become an expert quality management strategist; he offers his keen business acumen and superior quality management skills with an inclination to meet quality standards for the Hellenic Cord Blood Bank products at every stage. As a quality manager, he has not only maintained the utmost quality at the Hellenic Cord Blood Bank in processing and production, but has also created a number of policies and standard operating procedures to revamp outdated and lacking methods of production. He ensures that everyone is doing the best at every step of the procedure to achieve products of the highest quality. In 2012, and following specific and difficult training, Dr. Michalopoulos became an accredited inspector for the Foundation of Accreditation of Cellular Therapy and so far has inspected 12 cord blood banks globally. To date, he has published more than 30 articles, indexed in PubMed (MEDLINE), performed peer-reviews for journals, and has given lectures in conferences as an invited speaker.

Preface to "Modern Approaches in Cardiovascular Disease Therapeutics: From Molecular Genetics to Tissue Engineering"

Cardiovascular disease (CAD) is the leading cause of death globally out of all the non-communicable diseases. CAD is a group of complex disorders, which includes peripheral arterial disease, coronary heart disease, cerebrovascular disease, and rheumatic heart disease. Each year, more than 800,000 bypass surgeries are performed. Additionally, it is speculated that more than 17 million people have died due to CAD, representing approximately 31% of all deaths worldwide.

It has been speculated that CAD costs the European Union (EU) more than EUR 210 billion, and more than USD 300 billion in the case of the United States of America (USA) every year. The primary cause for the development of CAD is atherogenesis and developed atherosclerosis, which induces functional alterations to the vessels of the circulatory system. In this process, an individual's genetic background may influence the progression of this disease. Indeed, among other factors, genetic alterations regarding the function of immune cells and the human leukocyte antigen (HLA) system play a crucial role in the pathogenesis of CAD. An improved understanding of an individual's genetic alterations, which are specific for the initiation and progression of CAD, may facilitate the introduction of novel targets for advanced therapeutics.

Advanced approaches for CAD prevention also involve the use of suitable tissue-engineered vascular grafts (TEVG) for bypass surgeries. The gold standard conduits for this purpose are the Dacron- or ePTFE-derived vascular grafts. In addition, autologous grafts, such as the saphenous vein, have also been applied in the past. Unfortunately, less than 40% of patients have autologous vessels suitable for this purpose. Additionally, animal-derived vessels have been tested for their suitability as conduits. Recently, the production of TEVG using decellularization methods has gained significant attention from the scientific community. In the aforementioned approaches, the mechanical properties of the produced grafts are the main focus, and their study may reveal valuable information regarding their structure–function properties.

Modern approaches for CAD will take into account an individual's characteristics, promoting, in this way, advanced personalized therapeutic strategies in accordance with the conditions of good manufacturing practices (GMP).

We are delighted to present the current Special Issue, entitled "Modern Approaches in Cardiovascular Disease Therapeutics: From Molecular Genetics to Tissue Engineering". This collection of articles will involve the most relevant and state-of-the-art research related to the topic of the Special Issue, including, but not limited to, the following:

Molecular analysis of cardiovascular disease;
Novel biomarkers of cardiovascular disease;
Population genetics and association with cardiovascular disease;
Novel approaches for cardiovascular disease administration;
Vascular grafts and their application in cardiovascular disease;
Biomechanical properties of TEVG.

Panagiotis Mallis, Efstathios Michalopoulos
Editors

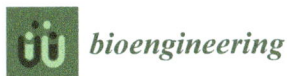

Editorial

Modern Approaches in Cardiovascular Disease Therapeutics: From Molecular Genetics to Tissue Engineering

Panagiotis Mallis *, Efstathios Michalopoulos and Catherine Stavropoulos-Giokas

Hellenic Cord Blood Bank, Biomedical Research Foundation Academy of Athens, 4 Soranou Ephessiou Street, 115 27 Athens, Greece; smichal@bioacademy.gr (E.M.); cstavrop@bioacademy.gr (C.S.-G.)
* Correspondence: pmallis@bioacademy.gr; Tel.: +30-210-6597340; Fax: +30-210-6597345

Abstract: Cardiovascular disease (CVD) currently represents one of the leading causes of death worldwide. It is estimated that more than 17.9 million people die each year due to CVD manifestations. Often, occlusion or stenosis of the vascular network occurs, either in large- or small-diameter blood vessels. Moreover, the obstruction of small vessels such as the coronary arteries may be related to more pronounced events, which can be life-threatening. The gold standard procedure utilizes the transplantation of secondary vessels or the use of synthetic vascular grafts. However, significant adverse reactions have accompanied the use of the above grafts. Therefore, modern therapeutic strategies must be evaluated for better disease administration. In the context of alternative therapies, advanced tissue-engineering approaches including the decellularization procedure and the 3D additive bioprinting methods, have been proposed. In this way the availability of bioengineered vascular grafts will be increased, covering the great demand that exists globally. In this Special Issue of *Bioengineering*, we tried to highlight the modern approaches which are focused on CVD therapeutics. This issue includes articles related to the efficient development of vascular grafts, 3D printing approaches and suitable atherosclerosis models.

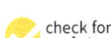

Keywords: cardiovascular disease; tissue engineering; small-diameter vascular grafts; mesenchymal stromal cells; 3D printing; decellularization; macrophages

---

Citation: Mallis, P.; Michalopoulos, E.; Stavropoulos-Giokas, C. Modern Approaches in Cardiovascular Disease Therapeutics: From Molecular Genetics to Tissue Engineering. *Bioengineering* **2021**, *8*, 174. https://doi.org/10.3390/bioengineering8110174

Received: 22 October 2021
Accepted: 3 November 2021
Published: 4 November 2021

Publisher's Note: MDPI stays neutral with regard to jurisdictional claims in published maps and institutional affiliations.

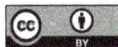

Copyright: © 2021 by the authors. Licensee MDPI, Basel, Switzerland. This article is an open access article distributed under the terms and conditions of the Creative Commons Attribution (CC BY) license (https://creativecommons.org/licenses/by/4.0/).

The development of functional vascular grafts, which can be applied in cardiothoracic surgeries, represents currently one of the greatest goals of tissue engineering. In particular, great effort has been made in order to better optimize the manufacturing procedures for the development of small-diameter vascular grafts (SDVGs) Globally, there is a great demand for this type of graft, applied mostly in coronary artery bypass grafting (CABG) [1,2]. Coronary artery obstruction represents one of the common manifestations of CVD [3]. CVD is a complex group of disorders, which involves peripheral arterial disease (PAD), coronary artery disease (CAD), cerebrovascular disease (CBD) and rheumatic heart disease (RHD) [1–4]. According to the World Health Organization (WHO), CVD is one of the leading causes of death globally, estimated to cause more than 17.9 million casualties each year [5]. The modern way of life such as daily diet, increased stress accompanied with high working hours and lack of physical exercise are the major factors that are related to the increased CVD occurrence [6,7]. Moreover, the proper management of CVD still represents a great burden from an economical point of view and on national health care systems, which are also characterized by major deficiencies in their daily routine [8,9].

The primary reason for CVD development is atherogenesis and developing atherosclerosis in the patient's vascular network [3,10]. In addition, an individual's genetic background plays a crucial role in disease progression. Therefore, the understanding of the underlying, associated pathogenetic factors may provide further insight for the better administration of CVD.

Currently, advanced therapeutic strategies are utilized in CVD patients, including the use of pharmaceutical regimens and modern vascular graft bioengineering applications [3]. To date, the gold standard procedure for the replacement of the occluded coronary arteries relies on the use of autologous secondary vessels such as the internal thoracic artery and saphenous vein [11]. In addition, fabricated vascular grafts made of synthetic materials such as Dacron and expanded polytetrafluoroethylene (ePTFE) have been applied in patients, although the success rate is variable [12]. Intriguingly, significant adverse reactions have occurred regarding the use of both strategies. Moreover, suitable autologous vascular grafts can be found in less than 30% of CVD patients, while synthetic SDVGs are characterized by a reduced patency rate (<60%) within the first year of application [3]. Other common manifestations include neointima formation and vessel occlusion, initiation of the calcification process and a severe host immune reaction [3]. These manifestations could lead to new vascular graft transplantation, which represents an unfavorable situation for the majority of the patients. Importantly, the application of synthetic SDVGs in pediatric patients is prohibited, due to their poor biological properties such as limited size alteration [3].

Therefore, and in order to avoid the aforementioned side effects, modern approaches in CVD must be evaluated as alternative therapeutic strategies. In this way, the application of advanced tissue engineering methods such as the decellularization protocol is currently being investigated for the potential SDVGs manufacturing [13–15]. The application of the decellularization method for the efficient production of SDVGs has gained attraction from the scientific community over the last decade [3]. Decellularization aims to produce an acellular biological scaffold through the removal of the tissue-resident cellular populations, while at the same time preserving adequately the extracellular matrix (ECM) [13–15]. The choice of the decellularization protocol is dependent on the tissue's origin and is necessary in order to produce a well-defined acellular scaffold. Utilizing the decellularization procedure, biological scaffolds can be efficiently derived from large animal models (such as porcine and bovine animal models), cadaveric donors, or discarded biological materials [13–15]. Besides the proper scaffold production, recellularization with host cellular populations must be performed in order to reduce any adverse reactions incidence. Taking into consideration the above, human umbilical arteries (hUAs) may represent a valuable alternative source for the production of functional SDVGs [16]. HUAs can be noninvasively isolated after gestation from the umbilical cord. Their inner lumen diameter ranges between 1–6 mm, and are characterized by three different wall layers (tunica intima, media and adventitia) and hence could resemble the structural function of human coronary arteries [16]. Additionally, animal-derived and biohybrid-fabricated vessels have been proposed [3]. However, the persistence of α-gal epitopes in decellularized scaffolds and the low biomechanical properties could limit their off-the-shelf application [17]. Additionally, advanced 3D bioprinting methods could enhance the SDVGs production process [18]. New bioprinting methodologies such as 4D printing will create a new era for the production of the next-generation (shape-shifted) vascular grafts [19]. In the near future, repopulated SDVGs with genetically engineered cellular populations, will be presented and used successfully in CVD patients, efficiently prolonging their lifetime. In the context of advanced approaches in CVD, the current Special Issue of *Bioengineering* aimed to gather modern studies related to translational vascular medicine. The current Special Issue included three original articles, two review articles and one editorial article.

The first article published by Mallis et al. [20] provided a comprehensive review regarding the fabrication of SDVGs and also the future perspectives, which will accompany their potent application.

Furthermore, Kozaniti et al. [21] presented the last evidence regarding the 3D printing approach and how can be associated with the production of functional vascular grafts.

Moreover, Garcia-Sabate et al. [20] developed a novel biomimetic 3D model to mimic atherosclerosis in order to investigate thoroughly the role of monocytes and macrophages in disease progression. Their work proved that the collagen density in the atherosclerotic plaque is the driving cause, thus inducing the secretion of specific adipokines and growth factors from the macrophages. The macrophage modulation mediated by the collagen density is further related to the atherosclerosis disease progression [22].

This Special Issue also involved an additional original research article prepared by Mallis et al. [23]. More specifically, this study provided evidence regarding the improvement of the repopulation methodology utilizing the cord blood platelet lysate (CBPL). In this study, the Mesenchymal Stromal Cells (MSCs) were dynamically seeded on decellularized vascular grafts. The performed histological analysis indicated the efficient repopulation of the vascular grafts with the MSCs. Indeed, vascular grafts treated with CBPL showed higher MSCs repopulation efficacy compared with the control group, as was determined by Ki67 and mitogen-activated protein (MAP)-kinase expression [23]. This proof-of-concept study indicated that the CBPL may improve the repopulation process, which may further reduce the processing time for bioengineered vascular graft production. Global research effort must be focused on the improvement of the functional vascular grafts manufacturing process. We hope that the current Special Issue of *Bioengineering* will motivate and inspire researchers of the field, worldwide. In this way, more data will be gathered, highlighting significant aspects which can be utilized in cardiovascular therapeutics, and in parallel improving the application of these advanced methods in terms of economics and quality.

Author Contributions: Conceptualization, P.M.; writing-original draft, P.M.; writing-review and editing, P.M., E.M. and C.S.-G.; supervision, P.M. and E.M.; Project Administration, P.M. and E.M. All authors have read and agreed to the published version of the manuscript.

Funding: This research received no external funding.

Institutional Review Board Statement: Not applicable.

Informed Consent Statement: Not applicable.

Data Availability Statement: Not applicable.

Acknowledgments: The guest editors of the current Special Issue want to express their gratitude to all contributors for their unique and outstanding articles. Additionally, special credits should be given to all reviewers for their comprehensive analysis and their overall effort in improving the quality of the published articles.

Conflicts of Interest: The authors declare no conflict of interest.

References

1. Zoghbi, W.A.; Duncan, T.; Antman, E.; Barbosa, M.; Champagne, B.; Chen, D.; Gamra, H.; Harold, J.G.; Josephson, S.; Komajda, M.; et al. Sustainable development goals and the future of cardiovascular health: A statement from the Global Cardiovascular Disease Taskforce. *Glob. Heart* **2014**, *9*, 273–274. [CrossRef]
2. Matters, C.D.; Loncar, D. Projections of Global Mortality and Burden of Disease from 2002 to 2030. *PLoS Med.* **2006**, *3*, e442. [CrossRef]
3. Pashneh-Tala, S.; MacNeil, S.; Claeyssens, F. The Tissue-Engineered Vascular Graft-Past, Present, and Future. *Tissue Eng. Part B Rev.* **2016**, *22*, 68–100. [CrossRef] [PubMed]
4. Abdulhannan, P.; Russell, D.A.; Homer-Vanniasinkam, S. Peripheral arterial disease: A literature review. *Br. Med. Bull.* **2012**, *104*, 21–39. [CrossRef]
5. World Health Organization. Available online: https://www.euro.who.int/en/health-topics/noncommunicablediseases/cardiovascular-diseases (accessed on 21 October 2021).
6. Noly, P.E.; Ben Ali, W.; Lamarche, Y.; Carrier, M. Status, Indications, and Use of Cardiac Replacement Therapy in the Era of Multimodal Mechanical Approaches to Circulatory Support: A Scoping Review. *Can. J. Cardiol.* **2020**, *36*, 261–269. [CrossRef]
7. Ditano-Vazquez, P.; Torres-Pena, J.D.; Galeano-Valle, F.; Perez-Caballero, A.I.; Demelo-Rodriguez, P.; Lopez-Miranda, J.; Katsiki, N.; Delgado-Lista, J.; Alvarez-Sala-Walther, L.A. The Fluid Aspect of the Mediterranean Diet in the Prevention and Management of Cardiovascular Disease and Diabetes: The Role of Polyphenol Content in Moderate Consumption of Wine and Olive Oil. *Nutrients* **2019**, *11*, 2833.
8. Maniadakis, N.; Kourlaba, G.; Fragoulakis, V. Self-reported prevalence of atherothrombosis in a general population sample of adults in Greece; A telephone survey. *BMC Cardiovasc. Disord.* **2011**, *11*, 16. [CrossRef]
9. Maniadakis, N.; Kourlaba, G.; Angeli, A.; Kyriopoulos, J. The economic burden if atherothrombosis in Greece: Results from the THESIS study. *Eur. J. Health Econ.* **2013**, *14*, 655–665. [CrossRef] [PubMed]
10. Lusis, A.J. Genetics of atherosclerosis. *Trends Genet.* **2012**, *28*, 267–275. [CrossRef] [PubMed]
11. Sanchez, P.F.; Brey, E.M.; Briceno, J.C. Endothelialization mechanisms in vascular grafts. *J. Tissue Eng. Regen. Med.* **2018**, *12*, 2164–2178. [CrossRef] [PubMed]

12. Ravi, S.; Chaikof, E.L. Biomaterials for vascular tissue engineering. *Regen. Med.* **2010**, *5*, 107–120. [CrossRef] [PubMed]
13. Gilbert, T.W.; Sellaro, T.L.; Badylak, S.F. Decellularization of tissues and organs. *Biomaterials* **2006**, *27*, 3675–3683. [CrossRef] [PubMed]
14. Gilpin, A.; Yang, Y. Decellularization Strategies for Regenerative Medicine: From Processing Techniques to Applications. *BioMed Res. Int.* **2017**, *2017*, 9831534. [CrossRef]
15. Crapo, P.M.; Gilbert, T.W.; Badylak, S.F. An overview of tissue and whole organ decellularization processes. *Biomaterials* **2011**, *32*, 3233–3243. [CrossRef]
16. Mallis, P.; Katsimpoulas, M.; Kostakis, A.; Dipresa, D.; Korossis, S.; Papapanagiotou, A.; Kassi, E.; Stavropoulos-Giokas, C.; Michalopoulos, E. Vitrified Human Umbilical Arteries as Potential Grafts for Vascular Tissue Engineering. *Tissue Eng. Regen. Med.* **2020**, *17*, 285–299. [CrossRef]
17. Macher, B.A.; Galili, U. The Galalpha1,3Galbeta1,4GlcNAc-R (alpha-Gal) epitope: A carbohydrate of unique evolution and clinical relevance. *Biochim. Biophys. Acta* **2008**, *1780*, 75–88. [CrossRef]
18. Jia, W.; Gungor-Ozkerim, P.S.; Zhang, Y.S.; Yue, K.; Zhu, K.; Liu, W.; Pi, Q.; Byambaa, B.; Dokmeci, M.R.; Shin, S.R.; et al. Direct 3D bioprinting of perfusable vascular constructs using a blend bioink. *Biomaterials* **2016**, *106*, 58–68. [CrossRef]
19. Gao, B.; Yang, Q.; Zhao, X.; Jin, G.; Ma, Y.; Xu, F. 4D Bioprinting for Biomedical Applications. *Trends Biotechnol.* **2016**, *34*, 746–756. [CrossRef]
20. Mallis, P.; Kostakis, A.; Stavropoulos-Giokas, C.; Michalopoulos, E. Future Perspectives in Small-Diameter Vascular Graft Engineering. *Bioengineering* **2020**, *7*, 160. [CrossRef]
21. Kozaniti, F.K.; Despoina, N.; Metsiou, A.E.; Manara, G.A.; Deligianni, D.D. Recent Advancements in 3D Printing and Bioprinting Methods for Cardiovascular Tissue Engineering. *Bioengineering* **2021**, *8*, 133. [CrossRef] [PubMed]
22. Garcia-Sabaté, A.; Mohamed, W.K.E.; Sapudom, J.; Alatoom, A.; Al Safadi Teo, J.C.M. Biomimetic 3D Models for Investigating the Role of Monocytes and Macrophages in Atherosclerosis. *Bioengineering* **2020**, *7*, 113. [CrossRef] [PubMed]
23. Mallis, P.; Sokolis, D.P.; Katsimpoulas, M.; Kostakis, A.; Stavropoulos-Giokas, C.; Michalopoulos, E. Improved Repopulation Efficacy of Decellularized Small Diameter Vascular Grafts Utilizing the Cord Blood Platelet Lysate. *Bioengineering* **2021**, *8*, 118. [CrossRef] [PubMed]

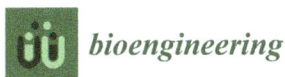

Article

Improved Repopulation Efficacy of Decellularized Small Diameter Vascular Grafts Utilizing the Cord Blood Platelet Lysate

Panagiotis Mallis [1,*], Dimitrios P. Sokolis [2], Michalis Katsimpoulas [3], Alkiviadis Kostakis [3], Catherine Stavropoulos-Giokas [1] and Efstathios Michalopoulos [1]

1. Hellenic Cord Blood Bank, Biomedical Research Foundation Academy of Athens, 4 Soranou Ephessiou Street, 115 27 Athens, Greece; cstavrop@bioacademy.gr (C.S.-G.); smichal@bioacademy.gr (E.M.)
2. Laboratory of Biomechanics, Center for Experimental Surgery, Biomedical Research Foundation Academy of Athens, 4 Soranou Ephessiou Street, 115 27 Athens, Greece; dsokolis@bioacademy.gr
3. Center of Experimental Surgery and Translational Research, Biomedical Research Foundation Academy of Athens, 4 Soranou Ephessiou Street, 115 27 Athens, Greece; mkatsiboulas@bioacademy.gr (M.K.); akostakis@bioacademy.gr (A.K.)
* Correspondence: pmallis@bioacademy.gr; Tel.: +30-2106597331 or +30-6971616467; Fax: +30-210-6597345

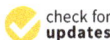

Citation: Mallis, P.; Sokolis, D.P.; Katsimpoulas, M.; Kostakis, A.; Stavropoulos-Giokas, C.; Michalopoulos, E. Improved Repopulation Efficacy of Decellularized Small Diameter Vascular Grafts Utilizing the Cord Blood Platelet Lysate. *Bioengineering* 2021, *8*, 118. https://doi.org/10.3390/bioengineering8090118

Academic Editors: Ngan F. Huang and Liang Luo

Received: 29 July 2021
Accepted: 24 August 2021
Published: 27 August 2021

Publisher's Note: MDPI stays neutral with regard to jurisdictional claims in published maps and institutional affiliations.

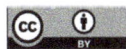

Copyright: © 2021 by the authors. Licensee MDPI, Basel, Switzerland. This article is an open access article distributed under the terms and conditions of the Creative Commons Attribution (CC BY) license (https://creativecommons.org/licenses/by/4.0/).

Abstract: Background: The development of functional bioengineered small-diameter vascular grafts (SDVGs), represents a major challenge of tissue engineering. This study aimed to evaluate the repopulation efficacy of biological vessels, utilizing the cord blood platelet lysate (CBPL). Methods: Human umbilical arteries (hUAs, $n = 10$) were submitted to decellularization. Then, an evaluation of decellularized hUAs, involving histological, biochemical and biomechanical analysis, was performed. Wharton's Jelly (WJ) Mesenchymal Stromal Cells (MSCs) were isolated and characterized for their properties. Then, WJ-MSCs (1.5×10^6 cells) were seeded on decellularized hUAs ($n = 5$) and cultivated with (Group A) or without the presence of the CBPL, (Group B) for 30 days. Histological analysis involving immunohistochemistry (against Ki67, for determination of cell proliferation) and indirect immunofluorescence (against activated MAP kinase, additional marker for cell growth and proliferation) was performed. Results: The decellularized hUAs retained their initial vessel's properties, in terms of key-specific proteins, the biochemical and biomechanical characteristics were preserved. The evaluation of the repopulation process indicated a more uniform distribution of WJ-MSCs in group A compared to group B. The repopulated vascular grafts of group B were characterized by greater Ki67 and MAP kinase expression compared to group A. Conclusion: The results of this study indicated that the CBPL may improve the repopulation efficacy, thus bringing the biological SDVGs one step closer to clinical application.

Keywords: decellularization; human umbilical arteries; mesenchymal stromal cells; repopulation; Ki67; MAP kinase

1. Introduction

The development of functional small-diameter vascular grafts (SDVGs), which can effectively be used in cardiovascular applications, remains a great challenge. Cardiovascular disease (CVD) represents a wide group of disorders, including peripheral arterial disease (PAD), coronary artery disease (CAD), cerebrovascular disease and rheumatic heart disease [1–4]. Changes in daily routine by adopting different behavioral habits, such as dietary change, smoking limitation and body exercise, may reduce the incidence of CVD [5–9]. However, CVD is one of the leading causes of death worldwide, estimating that more than 17 million people are suffering from some form of CVD [7]. In addition, more than 500,000 bypass surgeries are performed on CVD patients in the USA each year [10,11]. Therefore, the appropriate administration of CVD may result in a reduction in the corresponding global burden of death.

Different CVD cases require different therapeutic approaches, from medications' initiation to vascular graft replacement. Indeed, in the case of PAD and CAD, the utilization of vascular graft substitutes represents the most effective approach [12–14]. Currently, the gold standard approach for CAD is the replacement of the occluded vessel with another SDVG substitute [15,16]. Most times, secondary vascular grafts such as the saphenous vein and the mammary and radial arteries are preferred [16]. However, less than 50% of CVD patients are characterized by an adequate vascular network. It is known that CVD can cause significant hemodynamic differences throughout the whole patient's vascular network. In addition, accumulated atherosclerotic plaque in combination with stiffer blood vessels are common manifestations in CVD patients. Therefore, the utilization of suitable autologous secondary vascular grafts (e.g., saphenous vein), in order to be used for bypass grafting in those patients, is a demanding task [2,16]. As an alternative to autologous vessels, synthetic SDVGs can represent an important candidate [16]. The most used materials for vascular grafts fabrication are Dacron and ePTFE. Although synthetic vascular grafts made from Dacron and ePTFE have been used with promising results, in large diameter vessel replacement (e.g., aorta), their application as SDVGs is followed by severe adverse reactions by the host [17,18]. These adverse reactions may include the extended immune response against the synthetic vessel, platelet aggregation followed by clot formation, calcification development at the anastomoses sites, which further promote the graft rejection [17,18]. Moreover, the above-described adverse reactions may be deleterious for the patients and can even be life-threatening. Additionally, the use of synthetic SDVGs in pediatric patients is still not a favorable approach, unless there is no other alternative option [2,16]. In the past, also, cross-linked (formalin-fixed) vascular grafts of animal origin have been evaluated as vessel substitutes [19,20]. This type of grafts was characterized by totally different mechanical properties compared to the resident vessels, which could result in neointima formation and graft occlusion, due to compliance mismatch [16]. Moreover, formalin-fixed grafts have a limited in vivo remodeling ability; therefore, their potential application in CAD is reduced.

In the context of suitable SDVG development, the utilization of advanced tissue engineering approaches may guarantee an important solution to address the above issues [2]. In this way, the application of the decellularization method to produce SDVGs has been evaluated by various research groups worldwide [21–23]. Considering the above data, the potential use of decellularized human umbilical arteries (hUAs) has been proposed to be used as suitable SDVGs for CAD applications [21–23].

More specifically, the human umbilical cord (hUC) consists of two arteries and one vein [24–26]. The average length of the human umbilical cord can reach 50–60 cm [24,25]. The hUAs are responsible for the transportation of the non-oxygenated blood from the fetus to the mother. It has been calculated that more than 40 L of blood are transported through the hUAs. Histological analysis of the hUAs has revealed the presence of three layers in the vascular wall, the tunica intima (TI), media (TM) and adventitia (TA) [24,25]. Each layer is characterized by the presence of different cell populations, including the endothelial cells (in TI), the vascular smooth muscle cells (in TM) and the perivascular cells (in TA) [24–26]. In addition, hUAs are characterized by a lumen diameter of 2–6 mm and can be non-invasively isolated after gestation. Therefore, hUAs may represent an important candidate for the development of SDVGs.

To date, several research groups have evaluated the decellularized human umbilical vessels as vascular graft substitutes [21–23]. Decellularization aims to eliminate the vessel's cell populations, maintaining in parallel the integrity of the extracellular matrix (ECM) [26–28]. However, the repopulation of the vascular graft with host cells must be performed in order to gain its original functionality [29]. Most times, the proper repopulation (with the desired cellular populations, e.g., endothelial cells and vascular smooth muscle cells) of the decellularized vascular grafts is performed using vessel bioreactors under defined conditions [29]. However, the repopulation efficacy is still low; therefore, an improvement of the whole procedure may be considered. In such a way, the use of

CBPL may be applied as an additive to the repopulation process in order to improve cell adhesion. From advanced proteomic analysis, it has been shown that the CBPL contains a significant amount of growth factors including the platelet-derived growth factor (PDGF), transforming growth factor-β1 (TGF-β1), fibroblast growth factor (FGF), cytokines such as tumor necrosis factor-α (TNF-α), interleukin (IL)-1, IL-3, IL-6 and matrix metalloproteases [30–33]. The concentration and the combination of the above proteins have been shown to present tissue remodeling properties and also favor cell adhesion, proliferation and differentiation [34]. Currently, CBPL has been used widely in personalized regenerative medicine applications including wound and burn healing, and the regeneration of long-term skin ulcers in diabetic patients, while the standardization criteria for its proper production have also been described and published [35–37]. Therefore, the utilization of CBPL may improve the repopulation efficacy of the decellularized hUAs.

This study aimed to evaluate the impact of CBPL as a culture mediator for the improvement of SDVGs' repopulation. For this purpose, decellularized hUAs will be used as a potential scaffold for the repopulation experiments. MSCs derived from hUCs were seeded onto the decellularized hUAs and cultured in the presence of a cultivation medium containing CBPL. To evaluate the repopulation process, histological and biochemical analyses of the recellularized vessels were performed. The results of this study may deepen knowledge on efficient vascular graft development.

2. Materials and Methods

2.1. Isolation of hUAs

HUAs ($n = 60$, $l = 4$ cm) were isolated from the hUCs that were delivered to the Hellenic Cord Blood Bank (HCBB). All hUC samples were collected from end-term normal or caesarian deliveries (gestational ages 38–40 weeks) by experienced midwives. The informed consent for the enrolment of the current study was signed by the mothers before the gestation. The informed consent of the current study was in accordance with the ethical standards of the Greek National Ethical Committee and fulfilled the criteria of the Helsinki Declaration. The overall study was approved by the Bioethics Committee of BRFAA (No 2843, 7 October 2020). After the delivery to the HCBB, the hUCs were kept in Phosphate Buffer Saline 1× (PBS 1x, Gibco, Life Technologies, Grand Island, NE, USA) supplemented with 10 U/mL Penicillin and 10 µg/mL Streptomycin (Gibco, Life Technologies, Grand Island, NE, USA). The hUAs' isolation was performed within 24 h after the hUCs delivery. Briefly, the hUCs were rinsed in PBS 1x to remove the excess blood and blood clots. Then, isolation of intact hUAs was performed with the use of sterile surgical instruments. HUAs with occluded lumen were not used for the current experimental procedure and were discarded. Finally, each hUA was separated into two segments of 2 cm. The one-segment ($l = 2$ cm) was served as native hUA, whereas the other segment ($l = 2$ cm) was submitted to decellularization.

2.2. Decellularization of hUAs

The hUAs were decellularized based on an already published protocol from our research team [38]. Briefly, hUAs ($n = 60$, $l = 4$ cm) were placed in the first decellularization solution, which consisted of 8 mM CHAPS, 1 M NaCl and 25 mM EDTA in PBS 1x (Sigma-Aldrich, Darmstadt, Germany) for 22 h at room temperature (RT). Then, the hUAs were briefly washed in PBS 1x to remove the excess of the initial decellularization solution. After this step, the hUAs were placed in the second decellularization solution, which consisted of 1.8 mM SDS, 1 M NaCl and 25 mM EDTA in PBS 1x, (Sigma-Aldrich, Darmstadt, Germany) for another 22 h at RT, followed by a brief wash in PBS 1x. Finally, the hUAs were incubated in α-Minimum Essentials Medium (α-MEM, Sigma-Aldrich, Darmstadt, Germany) and supplemented with 40% Fetal Bovine Serum (FBS, Sigma-Aldrich, Darmstadt, Germany) for 48 h at 37 °C. All steps were performed under rotational and continuous agitation.

2.3. Histological Analysis of hUAs

The evaluation of the elimination of cellular populations and the ECM preservation in decellularized hUAs was performed with the histological analysis. Specifically, native (n = 5, l = 2 cm) and decellularized (n = 5, l = 2 cm) hUAs were fixed in 10% v/v neutral formalin buffer (Sigma-Aldrich, Darmstadt, Germany), dehydrated, paraffin-embedded and sectioned at 5 μm. Hematoxylin and Eosin (H&E, Sigma-Aldrich, Darmstadt, Germany), Orcein Stain (OS, Sigma-Aldrich, Darmstadt, Germany), Masson's Trichrome (MT, Sigma-Aldrich, Darmstadt, Germany) and Toluidine Blue (TB, Sigma-Aldrich, Darmstadt, Germany) were used for the evaluation of cellular/nuclear materials, elastin, collagen and sulphated glycosaminoglycans (sGAGs), respectively. Images were acquired with a Leica DM L2 light microscope (Leica Microsystems, Weltzar, Germany) and processed with ImageJ 1.46 r (Wane Rasband, National Institutes of Health, Bethesda, MD, USA).

2.4. Scanning Electron Microscopy Analysis of hUAs

Scanning electron microscopy (SEM) analysis was performed to further evaluate the ultrastructure of the hUAs. Specifically, hUA segments obtained from native (n = 5, l = 8 mm) and decellularized (n = 5, l = 8 mm). Then, all samples were initially fixed with 1% v/v glutaraldehyde solution (Sigma-Aldrich, Darmstadt, Germany). Briefly, rinses with distilled water were performed 3 times. Then, dehydration of segments was performed using 70% v/v, 80% v/v, 95% v/v aqueous ethanol and absolute ethanol for 20 min each. Dehydrated hUA segments were placed in hexamethyldisilazane solution (Sigma-Aldrich, Darmstadt, Germany) for 10 min, air-dried and sputter-coated with gold (Cressington Sputter, Coater 108 auto, Watford, UK). Finally, the samples were examined with SEM Phillips XL-30 (Phillips, FEI, Hillsboro, OR, USA).

2.5. Biochemical Analysis of hUAs

Collagen quantification of native (n = 10, l = 2 cm) and decellularized (n = 10, l = 2 cm) hUAs was performed with a Hydroxyproline Assay Kit (MAK 009, Sigma-Aldrich, Darmstadt, Germany), according to the manufacturer's instructions. Briefly, all samples were digested in 125 μg/mL papain buffer (Sigma-Aldrich, Darmstadt, Germany) at 60 °C for 12 h. Then, all samples were hydrolyzed with 12 M HCl, dried and incubated with Chloramine T/oxidation buffer and DMAB reagent. The hydroxyproline content, which corresponded to the collagen amount, was determined photometrically at 560 nm by interpolation to the hydroxyproline standard curve.

Accordingly, for the sGAG quantification, native (n = 10, l = 2 cm) and decellularized (n = 10, l = 2 cm) hUAs were digested in 125 μg/mL papain buffer. Then, in digested samples, the addition of dimethylene blue (Sigma-Aldrich, Darmstadt, Germany) was performed. Finally, the samples were quantified photometrically at 525 nm. The sGAG content was determined by interpolation to the standard curve (dilutions of 3, 6, 12, 25, 50, 100 and 150 μg/mL chondroitin sulfate were used for the development of the standard curve).

DNA quantification was performed in native (n = 10, l = 2 cm) and decellularized (n = 10, l = 2 cm) hUAs. To perform this quantification, all samples were digested in a lysis buffer that consisted of 0.1 M Tris pH 8, 0.2 M NaCl, 5 mM EDTA and 25 mg/mL Proteinase K (Sigma-Aldrich, Darmstadt, Germany), followed by incubation at 55 °C for 12 h. Inactivation of Proteinase K was performed after the complete tissue lysis, at 60 °C for 5 min. The DNA was isolated, cleaned and diluted in 50 μL of RNA-se-free water (Sigma-Aldrich, Darmstadt, Germany). Finally, the DNA amount in each sample was determined by photometrical measurement at 260 to 280 nm.

2.6. Preparation of hUAs for Biomechanical Analysis

Native (n = 10) and decellularized (n = 10) hUAs were analyzed for their biomechanical properties. Briefly, a ring-like (~1 mm width) and a strip-like sample (~5 mm long) were used for the qualitative histological observations. The hUAs (both native and decellularized) were cut into strips and ring samples along the circumferential and longitudinal direction, respectively. The occurred samples were placed in a Petri dish containing Krebs–Ringer solution at 37 °C. The frontal and the lateral aspects of the samples were observed under a stereomicroscope ((Nikon SMZ800; Nikon Instruments Europe BV, Amsterdam, The Netherlands) and images were acquired with a color digital camera (Leica DFC500, Leica Microsystems GmbH, Wetzlar, Germany). The inner and outer circumference, thickness, cross-sectional area and width of the ring and the strip samples were determined by measurements performed in the acquired images, using the Image-Pro Plus software (v 4.5, Media Cybernetics Inc., Bethesda, MD, USA).

2.7. Biomechanical Analysis of hUAs

For the biomechanical analysis of native ($n = 10$) and decellularized ($n = 10$) hUAs, an experimental device (Vitrodyne V1000 Universal Tester; Liveco Inc., Burlington, VT, USA) was used. The device consisted of (a) a stationary lower grip and an upper grip attached to the actuator, gradually extending the samples that were vertically mounted in the grips; (b) a load cell (GSO-250; Transducer Techniques, Temecula, CA, USA) with 0.01-g accuracy for the evaluation of load; (c) a rotary encoder providing feedback on the vertical displacement of the upper sample grip with 10-micrometer accuracy; (d) a saline bath wherein the samples were submerged during testing to sustain normal tissue hydration; (e) a heater coil (1130A, PolyScience, Niles, IL, USA) regulating the temperature of the saline bath at 37 °C; and (f) an accompanying personal computer, interfaced with the controller of the device via the Material Witness software package (v. 2.02, Liveco Inc., Burlington, VT, USA) to store the data. The ring and strip samples of hUAs were mounted in the device for the analysis, using hook-shaped grips. The unloaded length of all samples was obtained by vertically adjusting the upper grip to record only their weight. All samples were submitted to a progressively increasing tensile load at a 10 μm/s rate until full rupture of the wall.

2.8. Biomechanical Data Analysis

Stretch was calculated as the sample length during load increase by the experimental device (Vitrodyne V1000 Universal Tester; Liveco Inc., Burlington, VT, USA) divided by the unloaded sample length. The strain was calculated using the stretch values minus one. Stress was calculated by dividing the product of the load and stretch by their unloaded cross-sectional area, assuming tissue incompressibility. The stress–strain data were regressed with 9th-order polynomials, affording correlation coefficients $r > 0.95$, and the elastic modulus (tangent) at each strain level was calculated as the first derivative of stress over strain. Failure stress, representing tissue strength, and failure strain, representing extensibility, were calculated as the maximum stress and strain values at the first rupture. Peak elastic modulus, representing maximum tissue stiffness, was calculated as the highest elastic modulus value before the first rupture. All calculations were performed in Mathematica (v. 9.0, Wolfram Research Inc., Boston, MA, USA).

2.9. Quality Control of Isolated WJ-MSCs

MSCs used in this study were isolated from hUCs Wharton's jelly tissue, as previously described [31,39]. The quality check of the WJ-MSCs ($n = 5$) at passage (P)1-P3 involved (a) the determination of morphological characteristics, (b) performance of tri-lineage differentiation, (c) colony-forming units' (CFUs) assay performance and (d) immunophenotyping analysis using the flow cytometer.

The differentiation of WJ-MSCs into "osteocytes", "adipocytes" and "chondrocytes" was achieved using the specific kits according to the manufacturer's instructions. Specifically, the StemPro Osteogenesis, Adipogenesis and Chondrogenesis differentiation kits (Thermo Fischer Scientific, Waltham, MA, USA) were applied. To verify the differentiation efficiency of WJ-MSCs, histological stains were performed, as previously described [31,39]. For this purpose, Alizarin Red S, Oil Red O and Alcian Blue (Sigma-Aldrich, Darmstadt,

Germany) were used for the determination of calcium deposition, lipid droplet and sulfated glycosaminoglycans' (sGAGs) production, respectively.

CFUs assay was performed in WJ-MSCs at P1–P3. WJ-MSCs (from each passage) were detached from the culture flask using trypsin (0.025%)-EDTA (0.01%) buffer (Thermo Fischer Scientific, Waltham, MA, USA), counted, seeded at a density of 500 cells/well on 6-well plates and incubated for 15 days at 37 °C and 5% CO_2. Then, the cultures were washed with PBS 1x (Sigma-Aldrich, Darmstadt, Germany) and formalin-fixed. Giemsa stain was applied for 5 min, and the stained CFUs were observed under an inverted Leica DM L2 light microscope (Leica, Microsystems, Weltzar, Germany). In addition, the positively stained CFUs were microscopically counted by two independent observers.

Flow cytometric analysis was performed in order to determine the WJ-MSCs' immunophenotype, as has been proposed by ISCT [40]. For this purpose, 15 monoclonal antibodies (mAb) panel was used. This panel is composed of (a) fluorescein (FITC)-conjugated mAbs CD90, CD45, CD19, CD29, CD31 and HLA-ABC, (b) phycoerythrin (PE)-conjugated mAbs CD44, CD3, CD11b and CD34, (c) peridinin-chlorophyll-protein (PerCP)-conjugated mAbs CD105, HLA-DR and (d) allophycocyanin (APC)-conjugated mAbs CD73, CD10 and CD340. All mAbs were purchased from Becton Dickinson (BD biosciences, Franklin Lakes, NJ, USA). The immunophenotyping analysis was performed in FACS Calibur (BD biosciences, Franklin Lakes, NJ, USA) with at least 10,000 events at each tube. Flow cytometric data analysis was performed with FlowJo v10 (BD biosciences, NJ, USA).

For the below-described repopulation experiments, WJ-MSCs P3 were applied. In each passage, the total number and viability of WJ-MSCs were determined using automated count combined with trypan blue (Sigma-Aldrich, Darmstadt, Germany).

2.10. In Vitro Angiogenesis Assay

The ability of WJ-MSCs P3 to form networks was evaluated with the performance of an in vitro angiogenesis assay. Matrigel© (BD, Heidelberg, Germany) was thawed on ice overnight, according to the manufacturer's instructions. Then, 30 μL of the Matrigel© was placed in each well of 24-well plate and incubated for 30 min at 37 °C. WJ-MSCs P3, at a density of 3×10^4, were seeded into each well, followed by the addition of 500 μL of a-Minimum Essentials Medium (a-MEM) supplemented with Endothelial Growth Medium-2 (EGM-2). The networks were formed within 8 h. Images were acquired with a Leica DM L2 light microscope (Leica, Microsystems, Weltzar, Germany).

2.11. Repopulation of hUAs

For the repopulation experiments, Wharton's Jelly (WJ)-MSCs ($n = 5$) of P3 were seeded onto the decellularized hUAs. Quality characteristics of WJ-MSCs including immunophenotyping analysis, trilineage differentiation, proliferation potential (until P3) and viability assessment, were performed, as described in the previous section (2.9 Quality Control of isolated WJ-MSCs).

To perform the repopulation experiments, decellularized hUAs ($n = 10$) were cut into rings (l = 1 cm) and were placed in 15 ml polypropylene conical falcon tubes. Then, MSCs at a density of 1.5×10^6 cells were added to each hUA ring. Incubation at dynamic seeding conditions, using a thermal shaker, at 37 °C, for a maximum of 8 h, was performed. Then, the repopulated hUAs were placed into 6-well plates. The addition of WJ-MSCs P3 at a density of 1×10^5 cells in the 6-well plates was also performed. Finally, the 6-well plates containing the repopulated hUAs were placed into the incubator at 37 °C and 5% CO_2 for a time period of 30 days. Biweekly change of the culture media was performed to all repopulated hUAs. Repopulated hUAs were divided into the following two groups: group A—repopulated hUAs ($n = 5$) with WJ-MSCs P3 cultivated with regular culture medium consisted of α-MEM (Gibco, Thermo-Scientific, Waltham, MA, USA), 1% v/v Penicillin-Streptomycin (P-S, Gibco, Thermo-Scientific, Waltham, MA, USA), 1% v/v L-glutamine (L-glu, Gibco, Thermo-Scientific, Waltham, MA, USA) and 15% FBS (Gibco,

Thermo-Scientific, Massachusetts, USA and group B—repopulated hUAs ($n = 5$) with WJ-MSCs P3 cultivated culture medium consisted of α-MEM (Gibco, Thermo-Scientific, Waltham, MA, USA) supplemented with 1% P-S (Gibco, Thermo-Scientific, Waltham, MA, USA) and 15% v/v CBPL. The CBPL was produced based on a previously published protocol from our laboratory [30]. Briefly, for the production of CBPL, CBUs with an initial volume of 111–148 mL (including the anticoagulant) were used. None of the CBUs used for the production of CBPL met the minimum criteria of processing, cryopreservation and release outlined by the HCBB (Table S1). The CBUs were initially centrifuged at $210 \times g$ for 15 min at room temperature (RT). The top plasma fraction was transferred using a manual extraction system, to a secondary processing bag. The plasma fraction was centrifuged again at $2600 \times g$ for 15 min at RT. Finally, the supernatant platelet-poor plasma (PPP) was removed and the remaining CBPL (8–10 mL) was supplemented in α-MEM. Additionally, a sample obtained from CBPL was taken and counted in a hematological analyzer (Sysmex XS 1000i, Roche, Basel, Switzerland) to verify the platelet concentration within the CBPL. The culture media were used from the initial WJ-MSCs seeding onto the decellularized hUAs.

2.12. Histological Analysis of the Repopulated hUAs

The evaluation of the repopulation efficiency of the decellularized hUAs was performed with the histological assessment. Briefly, repopulated hUAs (from both groups) were fixed in 10% v/v neutral formalin buffer, dehydrated, paraffin-embedded and sectioned at 5 μm, as previously described. H&E staining was performed for the evaluation of the seeded WJ-MSCs onto the hUAs.

The proliferation potential of WJ-MSCs P3 in seeded hUAs was assessed by indirect immunofluorescence experiments. The primary antibody used in this experimental procedure was anti-MAP kinase, activated dephosphorylated ERK 1 and 2 antibodies (1:1000, Sigma-Aldrich, Darmstadt, Germany), while the secondary was FITC-conjugated anti-mouse (1:80, Sigma-Aldrich, Darmstadt, Germany) antibody. Finally, the sections were dehydrated, and glycerol was mounted. The images were obtained with an LEICA SP5 II confocal microscope with LAS Suite v2 software (Leica Microsystems, GmbH, Wetzlar, Germany).

Quantification of MAP kinase expression and DAPI staining in repopulated hUAs based on immunofluorescence staining was performed as has been previously published by Prasad et al. [41]. For this purpose, the Image J (v1.533, National Institute of Health, USA) was used. Specifically, the acquired figures were converted into 8-bit images and then, using the Split Channels tool, were split into their original images. Plot profiles of MAP kinase expression (FITC, green channel) and DAPI (blue channel) were generated using the Histogram tool. The generated graphs represented the mean fluorescence intensities (MFI) corresponding to MAP kinase expression and DAPI stain.

2.13. Statistical Analysis

Graph Pad Prism v 6.01 (GraphPad Software, San Diego, CA, USA) was used for the statistical analysis in the current study. Comparisons of total hydroxyproline, sGAG and DNA contents and morphometric data between all samples were performed with Welch's t-test. Comparison of DNA content and biomechanical results between all samples was performed with an unpaired non-parametric Kruskal–Wallis test. The statistically significant difference between group values was considered when p-value was less than 0.05. Indicated values were presented as mean ± standard deviation.

3. Results
3.1. Histological Analysis of hUAs

The impact of the decellularization approach in the ECM of the hUAs was evaluated using histological analysis. In this way, H&E, TB, MT and OS stains were applied in the native and decellularized hUAs for the evaluation of cell presence, sGAGs, collagen and elastin, respectively. The results of H&E indicated the absence of cell and nuclear remnants in the decellularized hUAs, while the ECM was adequately preserved (Figure 1). On the other hand, regarding the sGAG, a weaker stain intensity was observed in the decellularized hUAs (Figure 1). The collagen and the entire ECM were preserved in UAs after the decellularization, as it was indicated by an MT stain (Figure 1). In addition, OS confirmed the presence of elastin both in the native and decellularized hUAs. The histological analysis revealed that the decellularized hUAs were characterized by a more compact structure, compared to the non-decellularized native hUAs. Further histological examination of the inner structure and morphology of the hUAs was conducted using SEM analysis (Figure 2). The decellularized hUAs were free from their cellular populations (endothelial cells and smooth muscle cells, Figure 2). Moreover, SEM analysis revealed the successful preservation of ECM structures, thus further confirming the initial histological analysis (involved H&E, AB and MT stains).

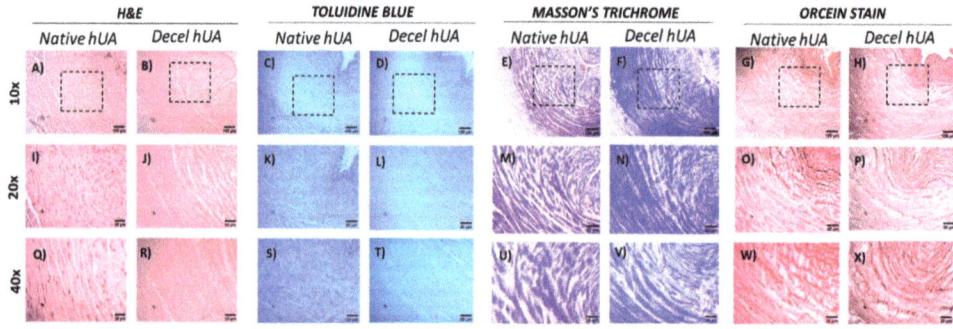

Figure 1. Histological analysis of hUAs (including native and decellularized samples). Native and decellularized hUAs stained with H&E (**A,I,Q** and **B,J,R**), TB (**C,K,S** and **D,L,T**), MT (**E,M,U** and **F,N,V**) and OS (**G,O,W** and **H,P,X**). The black boxes indicated the magnified field of 20× and 40× images. Images were presented with original magnification 10×, scale bars 100 µm, 20×, scale bars 50 µm and 40×, scale bars 25 µm. H&E: Hematoxylin and Eosin, TB: Toluidine Blue, MT: Masson's Trichrome, OS: Orcein Stain.

3.2. Biochemical Evaluation of hUAs

In the current study, DNA, hydroxyproline and sGAGs were quantified in order to properly evaluate the impact of the decellularization procedure on hUAs. Specifically, DNA was eliminated in decellularized hUAs. Specifically, the DNA content of the native hUAs was 1589 ± 150 ng DNA/mg of tissue weight. In the decellularized hUAs, the DNA content was 43 ± 6 ng DNA/mg of tissue weight, suggesting that 97% of the initial DNA content was removed (Figure 3A and Table S2).

Regarding the hydroxyproline (which corresponds to collagen content) content, no statistically significant difference was observed between the native and decellularized hUAs. The hydroxyproline content of the native and decellularized hUAs was 65 ± 9 and 61 ± 9 µg hydroxyproline/mg of tissue weight, respectively (Figure 3B). Finally, the sGAG content in the native and decellularized hUAs was 4 ± 1 and 2 ± 1 µg sGAGs/mg of tissue weight, respectively (Figure 3C). Statistically significant differences were observed in the DNA content ($p < 0.001$) and the sGAG content ($p < 0.01$) between the native and decellularized hUAs.

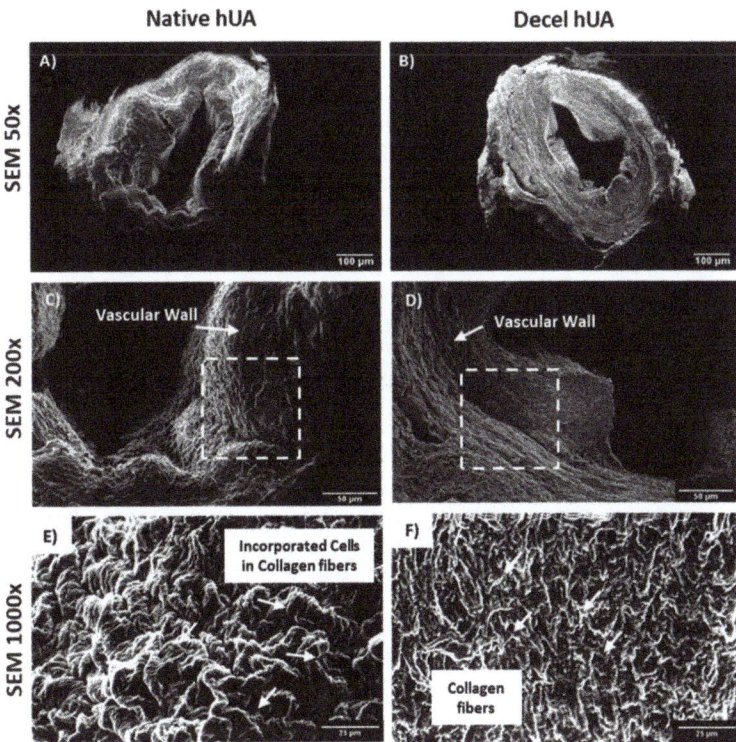

Figure 2. SEM histological analysis of hUAs. SEM images of native (**A,C,E**) and decellularized (**B,D,F**) hUAs. White arrows in images (**A,D**) represent the vascular wall. White squares in the same images represent the magnified region, as presented in images (**E,F**). White arrows in image E represent the combination of cells and collagen fibers of native, while in Figure **F**, white arrows represent only the preserved collagen fibers of decellularized hUAs. Images were presented with original magnification 50× (**A,B**), scale bars 100 μm, 200× (**C,D**), scale bars and 1000× (**E,F**), scale bars 25 μm.

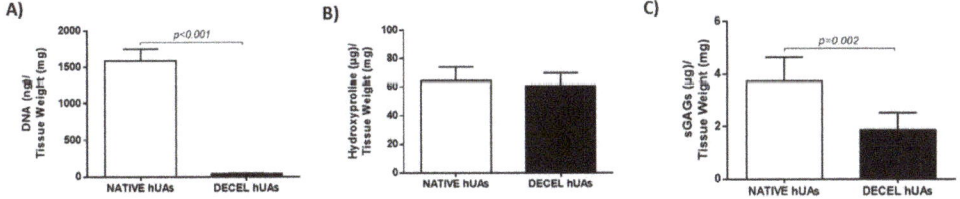

Figure 3. Biochemical analysis of hUAs. The biochemical analysis involved the DNA quantification (**A**), the hydroxyproline content (**B**) and sGAG content (**C**) quantification of native and decellularized hUAs. Statistically significant differences regarding the DNA ($p < 0.001$) and sGAG ($p < 0.01$) content were observed between native and decellularized hUAs.

3.3. Biomechanical Analysis of hUAs

The biomechanical properties of the native and decellularized hUAs were determined with the performance of uniaxial testing. In this way, both the native and decellularized hUAs were tested in longitudinal and circumferential directions. Regarding the longitudinal direction, the failure stress (σ), failure strain and peak elastic modulus for the native and decellularized hUAs were 755 ± 150 and 1373 ± 140 kPa, 1.4 ± 0.1 and 1.7 ± 0.2, 3458 ± 548 and 3867 ± 630 kPa, respectively (Figures 4 and 5A–C and Table S3). In the circumferential direction, the failure stress (σ), failure strain and peak elastic modulus for the native and decellularized hUAs were 1102 ± 180 and 1480 ± 150 kPa, 2.1 ± 0.3 and 2.7 ± 0.4, 3781 ± 540 and 5153 ± 420 kPa, respectively (Figures 4 and 5D–F and Table S3). Statistically significant differences regarding the longitudinal direction between the native and decellularized hUAs were observed in failure stress ($p < 0.05$) and strain ($p < 0.01$, Figure 5A–C). Regarding the circumferential direction, statistically significant differences between the native and decellularized hUAs were observed in failure stress ($p < 0.05$), failure strain ($p < 0.05$) and peak elastic modulus ($p < 0.05$, Figure 5D–F).

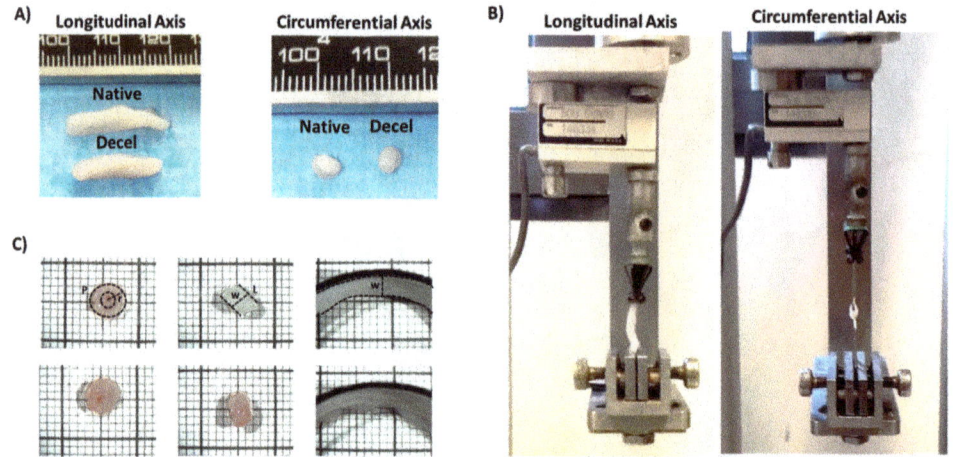

Figure 4. Set up of uniaxial biomechanical analysis of hUAs. Overview of decellularized hUAs in longitudinal and circumferential axis (**A**). Biomechanical testing of hUAs either in circumferential or longitudinal axis (**B**). Determination of hUAs dimensions using the stereoscope (**C**). P: Perimeter, r: radial, W: Width, L: Length.

3.4. WJ-MSCs Characterization

In this study, the WJ-MSCs P3 were applied for the in vitro recellularization of the decellularized hUAs. However, before further processing, the verification of the stem cell characteristics of the WJ-MSCs was performed.

The WJ-MSCs at P1–P3 presented a fibroblastic-like morphology. No change in their morphological features was observed between the passages (Figure 6A). The WJ-MSCs P3 differentiated successfully to "osteogenic", "adipogenic" and "chondrogenic" lineages upon stimulation with specific differentiation media. To determine the efficacy of the differentiation, histological stains were applied. Specifically, the mineral production (Ca^{2+} and Mg^{2+}) from the differentiated WJ-MSCs were determined with the performance of Alizarin Red S. Indeed, a high number of calcium deposits to the differentiated "osteocytes" were observed (Figure 6A). Moreover, successful CFUs development was performed by the WJ-MSCs from P1–P3 (Figure 6A). The corresponded CFU numbers developed by the WJ-MSCs at P1, P2 and P3 were 12.3 ± 1.6, 12.1 ± 1.5 and 13.1 ± 1, respectively. No statistically significant differences regarding the CFU number were observed between the different WJ-MSCs passages (Figure S1). Additionally, to verify the WJ-MSCs' properties to form an organized network, an angiogenesis assay was applied (Figure 6A). The WJ-MSCs started to develop the tubular networks after 4 h. An organized tubular network, formed by WJ-MSCs, was observed after 8 h of incubation.

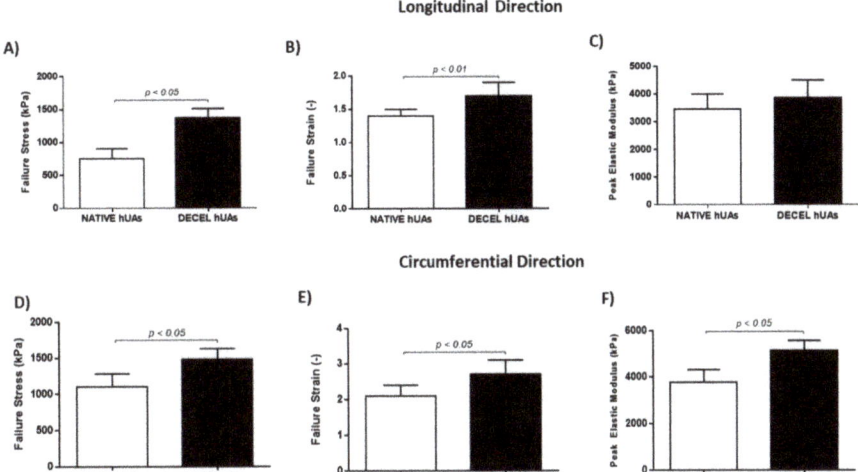

Figure 5. Biomechanical analysis of native and decellularized hUAs. Native and decellularized hUAs were tested for the maximum strain (**A,D**), failure strain (**B,E**) and peak elastic modulus (**C,F**), in the longitudinal (**A–C**) and circumferential (**D–F**) direction, respectively. Statistically significant differences between native and decellularized hUAs were found in failure stress ($p < 0.05$, in both directions), peak elastic modulus ($p < 0.05$, circumferential direction) and failure strain ($p < 0.01$ for the longitudinal direction and $p < 0.05$ for the circumferential direction). DECEL: Decellularized.

The immunophenotyping analysis of the WJ-MSCs P3 showed an expression >90% for the CD73, CD90, CD105, CD29, CD10, CD44, CD340 and HLA-ABC expression <2% for the CD3, CD19, CD34, CD45, CD15, CD11b, CD31 and HLA-DR (Figure 6B, Figure S2 and Table S4). Finally, the WJ-MSCs were expanded successfully since their first isolation until reached P3 (Figure 6C). Specifically, the mean number of WJ-MSCs at P1 was 1.8×10^6, at P2 it was 3.9×10^6 and at P3 it was 7.8×10^6 (Figure 6C). The viability of the WJ-MSCs at P1, P2 and P3 was $93.6 \pm 1.3\%$, $93.1 \pm 1.5\%$ and $93.3 \pm 1.3\%$, respectively, as confirmed by the trypan blue assay (Figure 6D).

3.5. Recellularization of hUAs

The WJ-MSCs P3 successfully repopulated the decellularized hUAs in both groups. However, a more uniform repopulation of the hUAs was observed when CBPL was used (Figure 7) Indeed, when CBPL was used as a supplement of the culture medium, a better distribution of the WJ-MSCs P3 was observed, compared to group A. H&E stain confirmed the presence of the WJ-MSCs P3 to the TA of hUAs in both groups (Figure 8). However, after 30 days of incubation, an extensive migration of cells from TA to TI was reported only in group B (Figure 8). The WJ-MSCs P3 of group A did not migrate, thus they were located only in the TA of the hUAs. Moreover, a greater number of the WJ-MSCs P3 were observed in group B compared to group A.

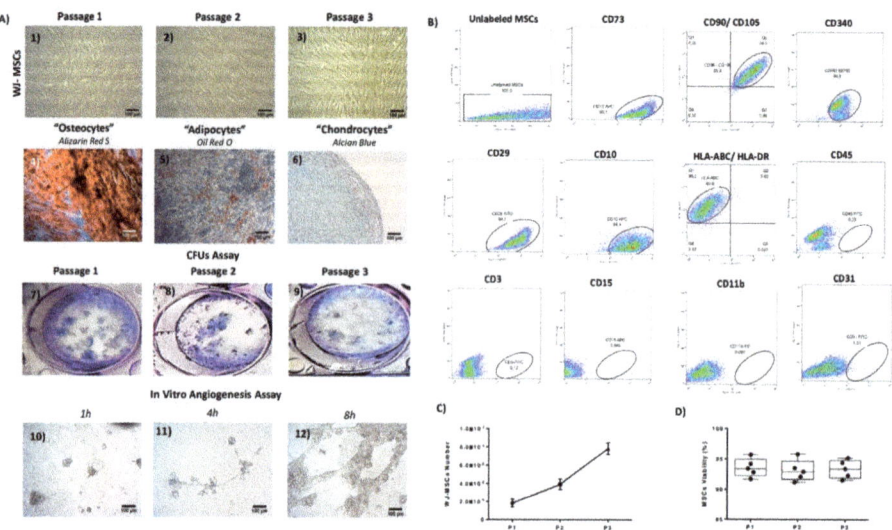

Figure 6. Characterization of the isolated WJ-MSCs. Morphological characteristics of WJ-MSCs (**A1–A3**). Differentiation of WJ-MSCs towards "osteogenic", "adipogenic" and "chondrogenic" lineages (**A4–A6**). The successful differentiation of WJ-MSCs into "osteocytes", "adipocytes" and "chondrocytes" was verified using the histological stains Alizarin Red S, Oil Red O and Alcian Blue, respectively. CFUs assay of WJ-MSCs at P1 to P3 (**A7–A9**). In vitro angiogenesis assay performance. Images showing the developed network were acquired after 1, 4 and 8 h (**A10–A12**). Immunophenotyping analysis of WJ-MSCs P3 (**B**). Determination of total number (**C**) and viability of WJ-MSCs at P1–P3 (**D**). The images **A1–A6** and **A10–A12** were acquired with original magnification 10×, and scale bars 100 µm.

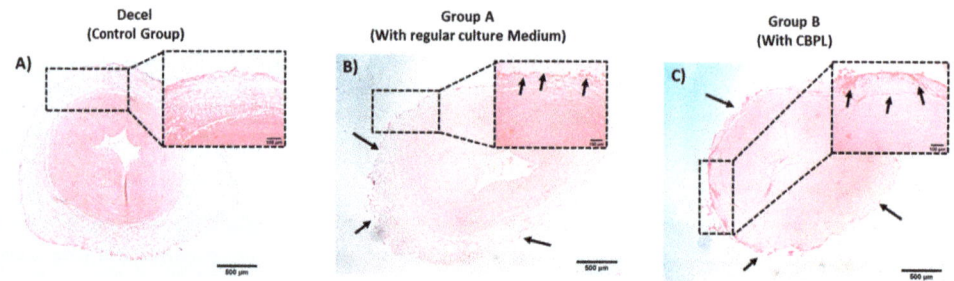

Figure 7. Histological analysis of hUAs (**A–C**). Overview of repopulated hUAs of groups A and B (**B**,**C**). Decellularized hUA served as the control group (**A**). Repopulated hUA of group A (**B**). WJ-MSCs P3 in group A were located only to the tunica adventitia. Repopulated hUA of group B (**C**). On the contrary, WJ-MSCs P3 in group B migrated successfully to the inner vascular wall. Images represented with original magnification 2.5× and scale bars 500 µm. Images in the black squares represented with original magnification 10×, scale bars 100 µm.

To further confirm the proliferative activity of the WJ-MSCs P3 in the repopulated hUAs, immunohistochemistry against Ki67 was performed (Figure 9). The expression of Ki67 was confirmed in both groups. However, a greater distribution of Ki67 was observed in group B, further confirming the H&E staining results.

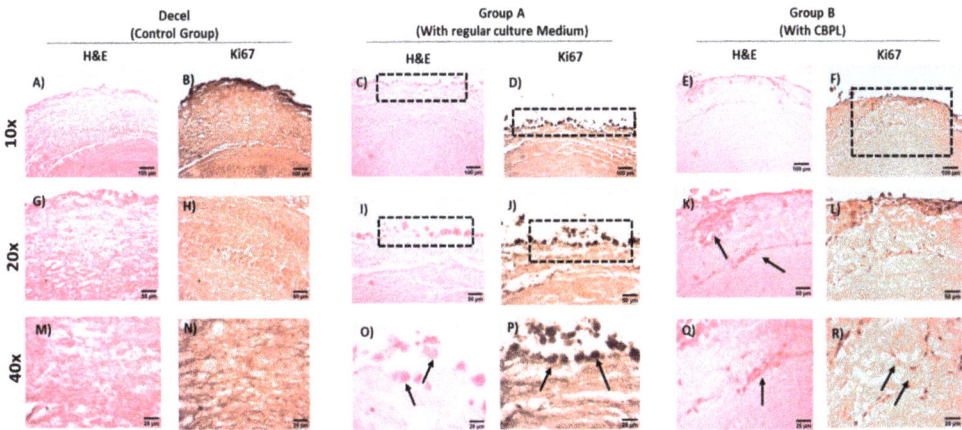

Figure 8. Histological analysis of repopulated vascular grafts with WJ-MSCs P3, located in the tunica adventitia. Decellularized hUAs stained with H&E (**A,G,M**). Repopulated hUAs of group A (**C,I,O**) and group B (**E,K,Q**) stained with H&E. Immunohistochemistry against Ki67 in decellularized hUAs (**B,H,N**), and repopulated hUAs of group A (**D,J,P**) and group B (**F,L,R**). Images (**A–F**) presented with original magnification 10×, scale bars 100 μm. Images (**G–L**) presented with original magnification 20×, scale bars 50 μm. Images (**M–R**) presented with original magnification 40×, scale bars 25 μm.

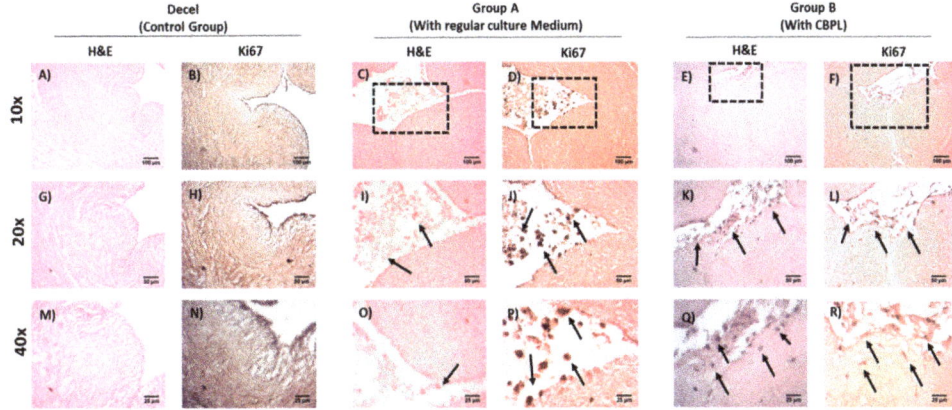

Figure 9. Histological analysis of repopulated vascular grafts with WJ-MSCs P3, located in the tunica intima. Decellularized hUAs stained with H&E (**A,G,M**). Repopulated hUAs of group A (**C,I,O**) and group B (**E,K,Q**) stained with H&E. Immunohistochemistry against Ki67 in decellularized hUAs (**B,H,N**), and repopulated hUAs of group A (**D,J,P**) and group B (**F,L,R**). Images (**A–F**) presented with original magnification 10×, scale bars 100 μm. Images (**G–L**) presented with original magnification 20×, scale bars 50 μm. Images (**M–R**) presented with original magnification 40×, scale bars 25 μm.

The immunofluorescence results indicated the expression of MAP kinase in both groups (Figure 10 and Figure S3). However, the greater distribution and expression of MAP kinase were observed in group B in comparison to group A (Figure 10). The MFI of the MAP kinase expression in TA and TI in repopulated hUAs of group A and group B was 13.9 ± 2.1 and 1.1 ± 0.3, and 45.6 ± 7.1 and 45.3 ± 5.1, respectively. Accordingly, for the DAPI stain, the MFI in repopulated hUAs of groups A and B were 7.6 ± 1.1 and 39.8 ± 2.5, and 43.4 ± 4.4 and 41.5 ± 4.3, respectively. The statistically significant differences were observed in the study groups, regarding either the MAP kinase expression ($p < 0.01$) or the DAPI stain intensity ($p < 0.001$). The latter further confirms the greater proliferative potential and migratory ability of the WJ-MSCs P3 in decellularized hUAs, when CBPL was also used as a supplement in the culture medium.

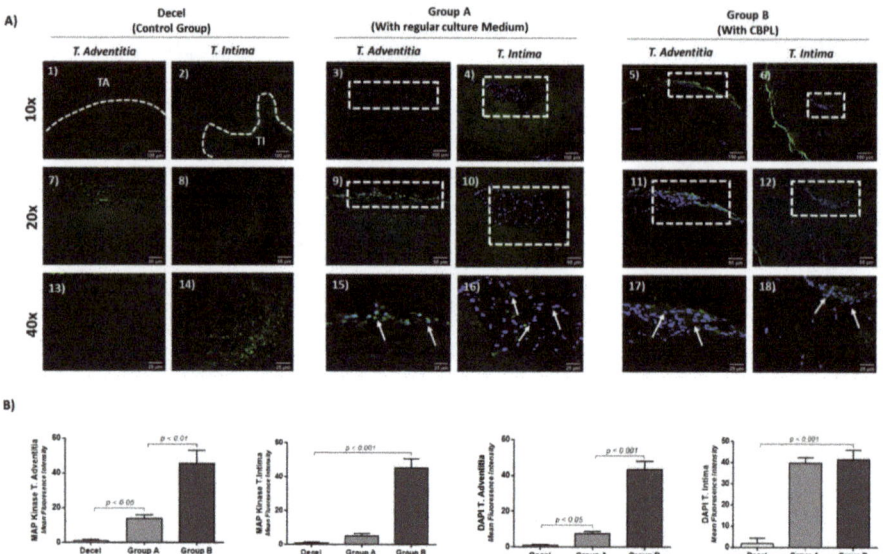

Figure 10. Indirect immunofluorescence against MAP kinase in combination with DAPI stain in repopulated hUAs (**A**). Decellularized hUAs did not exhibit any expression of anti-MAP kinase or DAPI stain (**1,2,7,8,13,14**) either in tunica adventitia or tunica intima regions. Repopulated hUAs in group A (cultured with regular medium) were characterized by both anti-MAP expression and DAPI stain (**3,9,15,4,10,16**). However, both signals were restricted only to the tunica adventitia of the repopulated hUAs (**3,9,15**). Repopulated hUAs in group B (with the use of CBPL) positively expressed the MAP kinase and DAPI stain both in tunica adventitia and tunica intima regions (**5,11,17,6,12,18**). Images (**1–6**) presented with original magnification 10×, scale bars 100 μm. Images (**7–12**) presented with original magnification 20×, and scale bars 50 μm. Images (**13–18**) presented with original magnification 40×, and scale bars 25 μm. Mean Fluorescence Intensity of MAP kinase and DAPI stain (**B**). Statistically significant differences regarding the MAP kinase expression and DAPI stain both in tunica adventitia ($p < 0.01$) and tunica intima ($p < 0.001$) in all groups. TA: Tunica Adventitia, TI: Tunica Intima. White boxes and arrows presented the presence of cells in repopulated hUAs.

4. Discussion

The fabrication of functional bioengineered SDVGs, suitable for CVD surgery, represents one of the major challenges of blood vessel engineering [15]. Current knowledge from the already performed research has shown that acellular SDVGs cannot be applied in patients due to severe host adverse reactions, such as thrombus and neointima formation [42,43]. In addition, decellularized animal vessels, cross-linked, sterilized, cryopreserved allografts or commercially available SDVGs fail to integrate properly to the damaged region [44–58]. Consequently, the host inflammatory response attributed by neutrophils and M1 macrophages is initiated, leading to platelet activation and aggregation [59]. Additionally, the cryopreserved allografts are characterized by increased bacterial infections [60]. In this way, the development of well-defined SDVGs requires further evaluation.

For this purpose, the repopulation of the decellularized SDVGs with host cellular populations may attenuate the aforementioned lethal consequences. The proper repopulation of the decellularized vascular grafts can be performed with the use of a suitable bioreactor system [61]. In this process, the optimum conditions for the repopulation of the grafts can be adjusted, ensuring the uniform distribution and proliferation of the cellular populations [62]. However, the whole process requires further improvement in order to reduce the fabrication time of the vascular graft.

In the majority of the studies, culture media utilizing FBS and synthetic growth factors are mostly applied [62–64]. FBS is a rich source of growth factors and hormones, which is commonly used as a culture media additive for the in vitro isolation and expansion of cells [65–68]. On the other hand, it has been shown, that significant variation in FBS content may exist between different lots [65–68]. Additionally, FBS may contain prions, xenogeneic antigens and bovine proteins, which can cause allergic reactions or the transmission of zoonotic diseases to the host [65–68].

Therefore, the utilization of better-defined supplements for the repopulation and fabrication of bioengineered SDVGs is an important asset. Previously conducted studies have shown that peripheral blood (PB) or cord blood derivatives, such as platelet-rich plasma (PRP) or platelet lysate (PL), may sustain the stem cell proliferation and, thus, can be used as an alternative to FBS supplement in the culture media [32,66–69]. Either PBPL or CBPL can induce the expansion of MSCs in great numbers, without altering their stemness properties [32,69]. CBPL has previously been used in combination with ascorbic acid for the development of vascular smooth muscle cells originating from MSCs [70].

The current study aimed to provide insight evidence regarding the beneficial use of CBPL in the repopulation of the decellularized SDVGs. For this purpose, the hUAs were decellularized effectively and served as scaffolds. Furthermore, WJ-MSCs were used as the cell population for the repopulation assays. As it has been shown previously by our group, hUAs can be efficiently decellularized, serving as an ideal scaffold for cell repopulation [39]. The preservation of the key specific ECM proteins in decellularized matrices, is of major importance, promoting the development of a suitable microenvironment for cell infiltration. In our study, the preservation of the ECM proteins was confirmed by the performance of the histological analysis. An H&E stain initially confirmed the preservation of an hUA ultrastructure, while at the same time no cell or nuclei materials were evident in decellularized vessels. Besides that, a more comprehensive analysis of hUAs' ECM involved the performance of TB, MT and OS. The above histological stains can specifically detect the sGAGs, collagen and elastin in the vessel wall of the hUAs. Indeed, MT and ES revealed the presence of collagen and elastin in the decellularized vessels in a similar way to the native ones. On the contrary, a weaker TB stain was observed in the decellularized hUAs, compared to the native hUAs, reflecting the possible reduction in the sGAG content. Moreover, the decellularized hUAs retained their initial collagen and elastin alignment to the vascular walls. This important finding has been related to improved biomechanical properties and better cell infiltration. The properly aligned collagen and elastin fibers retain their initial adhesion positions, which are important for cell infiltration, proliferation and differentiation. Indeed, these processes are mainly attributed by interactions between cell integrins ($\alpha 1\beta 1$, $\alpha 2\beta 1$ and $\alpha v\beta 1$) with the RGD binding motifs (arginine-glycine and aspartate), which are found in collagen and elastin fibers [71,72]. Similar results have been reported in the past by other research groups, thus further confirming the effective decellularization of the hUAs. Indeed, the successful preservation of fibronectin in decellularized hUAs, a protein that exerts important key-binding activities and has previously been shown by our research team [38,73]. Fibronectin, in a similar way as collagen and elastin, contains RGD binding motifs; therefore, mediated cell adhesion through integrins can be performed. On the other hand, decellularized SDVGs may need an additional pre-coating with heparin and VEGF in order to enhance the anti-coagulant properties and ECs' adhesion. Dimitrievska et al. [74] proposed a novel method for advanced heparin-binding in decellularized vascular grafts. This method is reliant on the covalent linking of high-density heparin in decellularized vessels, utilizing the "alkyne-azide" clickable dendrons. Furthermore, the same group showed that immobilized heparin induced a significant reduction in platelet adhesion, whereas the repopulation of the vessel with ECs was efficient. Koobatian et al. [75] showed that the addition of VEGF to the heparin binding domain may improve the long-term patency of the vascular grafts. VEGF favors the ECs migration and adhesion; therefore, a more uniform endothelium could be developed in the inner layer of the vascular grafts. Gui et al. [21] was the first who reported the efficient decellularization of hUAs and explored their potential use as SDVG. In this study, hUAs were decellularized, retaining their ultrastructure orientation in the same way as it has been reported in the current technical note. No discrepancies regarding the histological results were observed between the two studies. SEM images of native and decellularized hUAs further confirmed the production of a properly defined vascular graft. All the layers of the vascular wall (TI, TM and TA) were well preserved. No signs of ECM extensive destruction were observed in the decellularized hUAs.

Biochemical analysis of the collagen, sGAG and DNA content of the native and decellularized hUAs was performed in order to evaluate the decellularization process. The DNA content was eliminated in the decellularized hUAs. Additionally, the sGAG content showed a statistically significant decrease in the decellularized hUAs, compared to the native. On the other hand, the collagen content was preserved both in the native and decellularized vessels. The biochemical analysis results were in accordance with the histological stain observations. Indeed, the weaker TB stain in the decellularized hUAs was positively related to the loss of the sGAG content. At the same time, the absence of cell and nuclei materials confirmed the low DNA content in the decellularized vessels.

Due to the existence of variations between the native and decellularized hUAs, regarding the sGAG content and cell elimination, these may be related to the altered biomechanical properties of the decellularized hUAs. For this purpose, uniaxial biomechanical testing in longitudinal and circumferential directions was performed. Biomechanical differences were observed between the native and decellularized hUAs. These differences reflected the adaptation of a stronger and more extensible behavior in the decellularized hUAs compared to the native ones. Mostly, these differences existed only in the circumferential and not in the longitudinal direction. This alteration in biomechanical properties may be explained partially due to cell elimination and fiber disorganization. However, our histological analysis did not reveal collagen or elastin disorganization in the vascular wall of the decellularized hUAs. In addition, biochemical analysis revealed that decellularized hUAs were characterized by less sGAG content. Such alterations in the sGAG content, in combination with the loss of VSMCs, may cause the crimp of the collagen and elastin fibers. This, in turn, may increase the crosslink between collagen and elastin fibers, thus explaining the stiffer behavior of the decellularized hUAs. The presented biomechanical results were in accordance with previously conducted studies [76,77]. This may suggest that the decellularization may have an impact on the properties of the decellularized vessels.

Once the properties of the decellularized vessels were established, an evaluation of the repopulation efficacy with the WJ-MSCs with or without the CBPL was performed. Before the repopulation assessment, the WJ-MSCs were isolated, expanded and their characteristics were determined based on the ISCT criteria [40]. WJ-MSCs compromise a fetal stem cell population with unique immunomodulatory and regenerative properties [77–79]. It is universally known that MSCs are lacking the expression of HLA class II molecules, and co-stimulatory molecules (such as CD40, CD80 and CD86) [78–80]. Therefore, MSCs can be universally applied in the allogeneic setting of the tissue engineering approaches. Moreover, fetal MSCs (such as the WJ-MSCs) are characterized by longer telomeres and increased telomerase activity, and at the same time, by no mutations or epigenetic modifications to their genome, compared to the adult MSCs (such as the bone marrow or adipode Tissue MSCs) [78–83]. In addition, fetal stem cells can be greater expanded in vitro without any chromosomal instability [81–83]. Therefore, fetal MSCs may be a greater source of stem cells compared to adult cells for regenerative medicine applications. In the current study, it was shown that WJ-MSCs are capable of contributing to a vascular network formation, reflecting their ability to differentiate to other cells such as the ECs [78–83]. In the context of tissue engineering, a great number of easily handled cells is required for the successful repopulation of the decellularized matrices. In this way, the WJ-MSCs could represent a desired stem cell source for the successful production of functional SDVGs.

In the context of the repopulation procedure, WJ-MSCs P3 (with or without the addition of CBPL) were dynamically seeded to the decellularized hUAs for a time period of 30 days. Then, a histological assessment was performed. In both groups, WJ-MSCs P3 were successfully seeded in the decellularized vessels. However, the WJ-MSCs of group A were restricted only to the outer layer of the vessel. On the other hand, in group B, the WJ-MSCs were distributed more uniformly compared to group A. In group B, the WJ-MSCs were observed to migrate toward the TM of the vessel. Furthermore, the WJ-MSCs in both groups showed positive expression for Ki67.

To date, the PL mostly derived from the peripheral blood has shown promising results, regarding cell proliferation and differentiation in 2D conditions. Doucet et al. [84] indicated the better proliferation and expansion potential of MSCs cultured with PL compared to those cultured with fetal calf serum (FCS). Jooybar et al. [85] showed that PL can be used in various tissue engineering approaches. Specifically, Jooybar et al. [85] developed a novel injectable platelet lysate-hyaluronic acid hydrogel. Then, bone marrow MSCs were encapsulated in the aforementioned hydrogel. The results of this study indicated the high expression of *AGGRECAN (ACAN)*, *COLLAGEN I/II* and *SRY-BOX TRANSCRIPTION FACTOR 9 (SOX9)*. The encapsulated MSCs presented an increased metabolic activity and differentiation potential towards chondrocytes. Zhang et al. [86] showed the beneficial properties of PL regarding the neo-vascularization potential of decellularized rat pancreatic scaffolds. Indeed, the contained growth factors of PL supported the ECs' adhesion onto the decellularized pancreatic scaffolds. Finally, the repopulated scaffolds were implanted into the animal model. The results of this study showed that the released growth factors by the PL contribute significantly to better EC adhesion and vascular network development. The above pancreatic scaffolds were characterized by good biocompatibility, supporting, in this way, the long-term survival of the graft. However, until now, the CBPL has not been broadly applied in tissue engineering approaches. The current study represents a novel study, where the CBPL (with its contained growth factors) induced higher repopulation efficacy in decellularized hUAs, compared to the regular culture medium. In this way, CBPL may represent a better supplement for tissue engineering approaches, such as the production of functional bioengineered SDVGs.

Additional analysis of the repopulated vessels involved the detection of the dephosphorylated MAP kinase, using the immunofluorescence assay. Indeed, the WJ-MSCs in group B were expressed greater in the dephosphorylated MAP kinase, compared to group A. The monoclonal antibody (mAb), which was used, specifically recognized the activated MAP kinase isoforms ERK1 and ERK2. These isoforms are implicating in cell growth and proliferation [87,88]. It has been shown that ERK1/2 activation is required for the cells to move from the G0 to G1 phase, through the accumulation of phosphatidylinositol-3-OH kinase [89,90]. Accordingly, the overexpression of activated ERK1/2 in quiescent fibroblasts was sufficient to perform the S-phase entry [90]. Additionally, in loss of function experiments, using the PD98059 (an inhibitor of ERK1/2) observed a halt of the cell proliferation and growth factor production, which was acting with the tyrosine kinase receptors or G protein-coupled receptors in VSMCs [87,88]. Additionally, the use of another synthetic inhibitor (LY294002), specific for PI(3)K, blocked the DNA synthesis and the overall cell growth of cells [90–93]. This suggests that the activation of ERK1/2 plays a significant role in the downstream activation of other proteins such as PI(3)K, which contribute to cell growth and proliferation [90–93]. The activation of ERK1/2 can be promoted through the binding of various growth factors to their specific receptors. Among them, TGF-β1, VEGF, PDGF and FGF induce mitogenic benefits to cells through the activation of MAK isoforms [94–97]. Previous studies, conducted by our research team and also by others, have shown that CBPL is characterized by significant growth factor content [30,31]. TGF-β1, FGF, VEGF, PDGF, IGF, cytokines and chemokines are represented in the CBPL. In this way, it could be explained that repopulated vessels with CBPL were characterized by high WJ-MSCs proliferation and distribution to the vascular wall.

5. Conclusions

The current study described, in detail, the impact of the decellularization procedure to the vessels and the repopulation efficacy using the CBPL. CBPL, as a supplement to the culture media, may significantly improve the repopulation process. The future goal of our research will be the use of the CBPL culture medium in a vessel bioreactor system in order to assess if the proposed medium produced better-cellularized vessels. The utilization of

CBPL may add more beneficial properties to the repopulated vessels, avoiding, in this way, any allergic reactions from the host. In turn, this may bring the production of fully personalized vascular grafts one step closer to clinical utility.

Supplementary Materials: The following are available online at https://www.mdpi.com/article/10.3390/bioengineering8090118/s1. Figure S1. WJ-MSCs CFUs counting. No statistically significant differences were observed between WJ-MSCs at P1–P3. Figure S2. Flow Cytometric analysis of WJ-MSCs P3. High (A) and low (B) expression of CDs in WJ-MSCs P3. Figure S3. Indirect immunofluorescence against MAP kinase in combination with DAPI stain in repopulated hUAs. Indirect immunofluorescence of decel hUAs (A, B, G, H, M, N), group A (C, D, I, J, O, P) and group B (E, F, K, L, Q, R). Images A-R, presented with original magnification 40×, scale bars 25 μm. Table S1. Acceptable range of results outlined by the HCBB for processing and storage of cord blood units. Table S2. Raw data of DNA quantification. Table S3. Biomechanical analysis of native and decellularized hUAs. Statistically significant differences between the samples of longitudinal and circumferential direction were observed in failure stress (p< 0.01). Table S4. Flow Cytometric analysis of WJ-MSCs P3.

Author Contributions: Conceptualization, P.M., C.S.-G. and E.M.; validation, P.M., M.K. and D.P.S.; investigation, P.M., D.P.S. and M.K.; data curation, P.M., D.P.S., M.K. and E.M.; writing—original draft preparation, P.M., writing—review and editing, P.M., M.K., E.M. and D.P.S.; supervision, E.M., A.K. and C.S.-G.; project administration, E.M. and C.S.-G. All authors have read and agreed to the published version of the manuscript.

Funding: This research co-financed by the European Union and Greek National Funds through the Operational Program Competitiveness, Entrepreneurship and Innovation, under the call RESEARCH-CREATE-INNOVATE (project code: T1EDK-05722).

Institutional Review Board Statement: The current study was approved by the Bioethics Committee of BRFAA (No 2843, 7 October 2020).

Informed Consent Statement: Informed consent was signed and obtained from the mothers before the gestation. The informed consent was in accordance with the ethical standards of the Greek National Ethical Committee and fulfilled the criteria of the Helsinki Declaration.

Data Availability Statement: Not applicable.

Conflicts of Interest: The authors declare no conflict of interest.

References

1. Suglia, S.F.; Appleton, A.A.; Bleil, M.E.; Campo, R.A.; Dube, S.R.; Fagundes, C.P.; Heard-Garris, N.J.; Johnson, S.B.; Slopen, N.; Stoney, C.M.; et al. Timing, duration, and differential susceptibility to early life adversities and cardiovascular disease risk across the lifespan: Implications for future research. *Prev. Med.* **2021**, *153*, 106736. [CrossRef]
2. Mallis, P.; Kostakis, A.; Stavropoulos-Giokas, C.; Michalopoulos, E. Future Perspectives in Small-Diameter Vascular Graft Engineering. *Bioengineering* **2020**, *7*, 160. [CrossRef]
3. Zoghbi, W.A.; Duncan, T.; Antman, E.; Barbosa, M.; Champagne, B.; Chen, D.; Gamra, H.; Harold, J.G.; Josephson, S.; Komajda, M.; et al. Sustainable development goals and the future of cardiovascular health: A statement from the Global Cardiovascular Disease Taskforce. *Glob. Heart.* **2014**, *9*, 273–274. [CrossRef]
4. Abdulhannan, P.; Russell, D.; Homer-Vanniasinkam, S. Peripheral arterial disease: A literature review. *Br. Med. Bull.* **2012**, *104*, 21–39. [CrossRef] [PubMed]
5. Noly, P.-E.; Ali, W.B.; Lamarche, Y.; Carrier, M. Status, Indications, and Use of Cardiac Replacement Therapy in the Era of Multimodal Mechanical Approaches to Circulatory Support: A Scoping Review. *Can. J. Cardiol.* **2019**, *36*, 261–269. [CrossRef] [PubMed]
6. Ditano-Vázquez, P.; Torres-Peña, J.D.; Galeano-Valle, F.; Pérez-Caballero, A.I.; Demelo-Rodríguez, P.; Lopez-Miranda, J.; Katsiki, N.; Lista, F.J.D.; Alvarez-Sala-Walther, L.A. The Fluid Aspect of the Mediterranean Diet in the Prevention and Management of Cardiovascular Disease and Diabetes: The Role of Polyphenol Content in Moderate Consumption of Wine and Olive Oil. *Nutrients* **2019**, *11*, 2833. [CrossRef]
7. World Health Organization Cardiovascular Diseases (CVDs). Available online: https://www.who.int/news-room/fact-sheets/detail/cardiovascular-diseases-(cvds) (accessed on 25 October 2020).
8. Maniadakis, N.; Kourlaba, G.; Fragoulakis, V. Self-Reported prevalence of atherothrombosis in a general population sample of adults in Greece; A telephone survey. *BMC Cardiovasc. Disord.* **2011**, *11*, 16. [CrossRef]
9. Maniadakis, N.; Kourlaba, G.; Angeli, A.; Kyriopoulos, J. The economic burden if atherothrombosis in Greece: Results from the THESIS study. *Eur. J. Health Econ.* **2013**, *14*, 655–665. [CrossRef]

10. Mensah, G.A.; Brown, D.W. An Overview Of Cardiovascular Disease Burden In The United States. *Health Aff.* **2007**, *26*, 38–48. [CrossRef] [PubMed]
11. Heart and Stroke Statistics. Available online: https://www.heart.org/en/about-us/heart-and-stroke-association-statistics (accessed on 25 October 2020).
12. Dimeling, G.; Bakaeen, L.; Khatri, J.; Bakaeen, F.G. CABG: When, why, and how? *Cleve Clin. J. Med.* **2021**, *88*, 295–303. [CrossRef] [PubMed]
13. McGah, P.M.; Leotta, D.F.; Beach, K.W.; Zierler, R.E.; Riley, J.J.; Aliseda, A. Hemodynamic conditions in a failing peripheral artery bypass graft. *J. Vasc. Surg.* **2012**, *56*, 403–409. [CrossRef]
14. Fazal, F.; Raghav, S.; Callanan, A.; Koutsos, V.; Radacsi, N. Recent advancements in the bioprinting of vascular grafts. *Biofabrication* **2021**, *13*, 032003. [CrossRef] [PubMed]
15. Nugent, H.M.; Edelman, E.R. Tissue engineering therapy for cardiovascular disease. *Circ. Res.* **2003**, *92*, 1068–1078. [CrossRef]
16. Pashneh-Tala, S.; MacNeil, S.; Claeyssens, F. The Tissue-Engineered Vascular Graft-Past, Present, and Future. *Tissue Eng. Part B Rev.* **2016**, *22*, 68–100. [CrossRef]
17. Lodi, M.; Cavallini, G.; Susa, A.; Lanfredi, M. Biomaterials and immune system: Cellular reactivity towards PTFE and Dacron vascular substitutes pointed out by the leukocyte adherence inhibition (LAI) test. *Int. Angiol.* **1988**, *7*, 344–348.
18. Mitchell, R.N. Graft Vascular Disease: Immune Response Meets the Vessel Wall. *Annu. Rev. Pathol. Mech. Dis.* **2009**, *4*, 19–47. [CrossRef]
19. Liu, Z.; Zhu, B.; Wang, X.; Jing, Y.; Wang, P.; Wang, S.; Xu, H. Clinical studies of hemodialysis access through formaldehyde-fixed arterial allografts. *Kidney Int.* **2007**, *72*, 1249–1254. [CrossRef]
20. Canaud, B. Formaldehyde-Fixed arterial allograft as a novel vascular access alternative in end-stage renal disease patients. *Kidney Int.* **2007**, *72*, 1179–1181. [CrossRef]
21. Gui, L.; Muto, A.; Chan, S.A.; Breuer, C.; Niklason, L.E. Development of Decellularized Human Umbilical Arteries as Small-Diameter Vascular Grafts. *Tissue Eng. Part. A* **2009**, *15*, 2665–2676. [CrossRef]
22. Kerdjoudj, H.; Berthelemy, N.; Rinckenbach, S.; Kearney-Schwartz, A.; Montagne, K.; Schaaf, P.; Lacolley, P.; Stoltz, J.-F.; Voegel, J.-C.; Menu, P. Small Vessel Replacement by Human Umbilical Arteries With Polyelectrolyte Film-Treated Arteries: In Vivo Behavior. *J. Am. Coll. Cardiol.* **2008**, *52*, 1589–1597. [CrossRef]
23. Porzionato, A.; Stocco, E.; Barbon, S.; Grandi, F.; Macchi, V.; De Caro, R. Tissue-Engineered Grafts from Human Decellularized Extracellular Matrices: A Systematic Review and Future Perspectives. *Int. J. Mol. Sci.* **2018**, *19*, 4117. [CrossRef]
24. Asmussen, I.; Kjeldsen, K. Intimal ultrastructure of human umbilical arteries. Observations on arteries from newborn children of smoking and nonsmoking mothers. *Circ. Res.* **1975**, *36*, 579–589. [CrossRef] [PubMed]
25. Longo, L.D.; Reynolds, L.P. Some historical aspects of understanding placental development, structure and function. *Int. J. Dev. Biol.* **2010**, *54*, 237–255. [CrossRef] [PubMed]
26. Crapo, P.M.; Gilbert, T.; Badylak, S.F. An overview of tissue and whole organ decellularization processes. *Biomaterials* **2011**, *32*, 3233–3243. [CrossRef] [PubMed]
27. Gilbert, T.; Sellaro, T.L.; Badylak, S.F. Decellularization of tissues and organs. *Biomaterials* **2006**, *27*, 3675–3683. [CrossRef] [PubMed]
28. Mozafari, M.; Yoo, J.J. Decellularization and recellularization strategies for translational medicine. *Methods* **2019**, *171*, 1–2. [CrossRef]
29. Scarritt, M.E.; Pashos, N.C.; Bunnell, B.A. A review of cellularization strategies for tissue engineering of whole organs. *Front. Bioeng. Biotechnol.* **2015**, *3*, 43. [CrossRef]
30. Mallis, P.; Gontika, I.; Dimou, Z.; Panagouli, E.; Zoidakis, J.; Makridakis, M.; Vlahou, A.; Georgiou, E.; Gkioka, V.; Stavropoulos-Giokas, C.; et al. Short Term Results of Fibrin Gel Obtained from Cord Blood Units: A Preliminary in Vitro Study. *Bioengineering* **2019**, *6*, 66. [CrossRef]
31. Christou, I.; Mallis, P.; Michalopoulos, E.; Chatzistamatiou, T.; Mermelekas, G.; Zoidakis, J.; Vlahou, A.; Stavropoulos-Giokas, C. Evaluation of Peripheral Blood and Cord Blood Platelet Lysates in Isolation and Expansion of Multipotent Mesenchymal Stromal Cells. *Bioengineering* **2018**, *5*, 19. [CrossRef]
32. Longo, V.; Rebulla, P.; Pupella, S.; Zolla, L.; Rinalducci, S. Proteomic characterization of platelet gel releasate from adult peripheral and cord blood. *Proteom. Clin. Appl.* **2016**, *10*, 870–882. [CrossRef]
33. Cáceres, M.; Hidalgo, R.; Sanz, A.; Martínez, J.; Riera, P.; Smith, P.C. Effect of Platelet-Rich Plasma on Cell Adhesion, Cell Migration, and Myofibroblastic Differentiation in Human Gingival Fibroblasts. *J. Periodontol.* **2008**, *79*, 714–720. [CrossRef] [PubMed]
34. Rebulla, P.; Pupella, S.; Santodirocco, M.; Greppi, N.; Villanova, I.; Buzzi, M.; De Fazio, N.; Grazzini, G.; Argiolas, M.; Bergamaschi, P.; et al. Multicentre standardisation of a clinical grade procedure for the preparation of allogeneic platelet concentrates from umbilical cord blood. *Blood Transfus.* **2015**, *14*, 1–7. [CrossRef]
35. Gelmetti, A.; Greppi, N.; Guez, S.; Grassi, F.; Rebulla, P.; Tadini, G. Cord blood platelet gel for the treatment of inherited epidermolysis bullosa. *Transfus. Apher. Sci.* **2018**, *57*, 370–373. [CrossRef]
36. Tadini, G.; Guez, S.; Pezzani, L.; Marconi, M.; Greppi, N.; Manzoni, F.; Rebulla, P.; Esposito, S. Preliminary evaluation of cord blood platelet gel for the treatment of skin lesions in children with dystrophic epidermolysis bullosa. *Blood Transfus.* **2015**, *13*, 153–158. [PubMed]

37. Mallis, P.; Michalopoulos, E.; Panagouli, E.; Dimou, Z.; Sarri, E.; Georgiou, E.; Gkioka, V.; Stavropoulos-Giokas, C. Selection Criteria of Cord Blood Units for Platelet Gel Production: Proposed Directions from Hellenic Cord Blood Bank. Comment on Mallis et al. Short Term Results of Fibrin Gel Obtained from Cord Blood Units: A Preliminary in Vitro Study. *Bioengineering* **2021**, *6*, 66. *Bioengineering* **2021**, *8*, 53. [CrossRef]
38. Mallis, P.; Katsimpoulas, M.; Kostakis, A.; Dipresa, D.; Korossis, S.; Papapanagiotou, A.; Kassi, E.; Stavropoulos-Giokas, C.; Michalopoulos, E. Vitrified Human Umbilical Arteries as Potential Grafts for Vascular Tissue Engineering. *Tissue Eng. Regen. Med.* **2020**, *17*, 285–299. [CrossRef]
39. Chatzistamatiou, T.K.; Papassavas, A.C.; Michalopoulos, E.; Gamaloutsos, C.; Mallis, P.; Gontika, I.; Panagouli, E.; Koussoulakos, S.L.; Stavropoulos-Giokas, C. Optimizing isolation culture and freezing methods to preserve Wharton's jelly's mesenchymal stem cell (MSC) properties: An MSC banking protocol validation for the Hellenic Cord Blood Bank. *Transfusion* **2014**, *54*, 3108–3120. [CrossRef]
40. Dominici, M.; Le Blanc, K.; Mueller, I.; Slaper-Cortenbach, I.; Marini, F.; Krause, D.; Deans, R.; Keating, A.; Prockop, D.; Horwitz, E. Minimal criteria for defining multipotent mesenchymal stromal cells. The International Society for Cellular Therapy position statement. *Cytotherapy* **2006**, *8*, 315–317. [CrossRef]
41. Prasad, C.P.; Chaurasiya, S.K.; Axelsson, L.; Andersson, T. WNT-5A triggers Cdc42 activation leading to an ERK1/2 dependent decrease in MMP9 activity and invasive migration of breast cancer cells. *Mol Oncol.* **2013**, *7*, 870–883. [CrossRef]
42. Kakisis, J.D.; Liapis, C.; Breuer, C.; Sumpio, B.E. Artificial blood vessel: The Holy Grail of peripheral vascular surgery. *J. Vasc. Surg.* **2005**, *41*, 349–354. [CrossRef] [PubMed]
43. Hamilos, M.; Petousis, S.; Parthenakis, F. Interaction between platelets and endothelium: From pathophysiology to new therapeutic options. *Cardiovasc. Diagn. Ther.* **2018**, *8*, 568–580. [CrossRef]
44. Gu, L.; Shan, T.; Ma, Y.-X.; Tay, F.R.; Niu, L. Novel Biomedical Applications of Crosslinked Collagen. *Trends Biotechnol.* **2019**, *37*, 464–491. [CrossRef] [PubMed]
45. Gough, J.E.; Scotchford, C.A.; Downes, S. Cytotoxicity of glutaraldehyde crosslinked collagen/poly(vinyl alcohol) films is by the mechanism of apoptosis. *J. Biomed. Mater. Res.* **2002**, *61*, 121–130. [CrossRef]
46. Elomaa, L.; Yang, Y.P. Additive Manufacturing of Vascular Grafts and Vascularized Tissue Constructs. *Tissue Eng. Part B Rev.* **2017**, *23*, 436–450. [CrossRef]
47. Brinkman, W.T.; Nagapudi, K.; Thomas, B.S.; Chaikof, E.L. Photo-Cross-Linking of Type I Collagen Gels in the Presence of Smooth Muscle Cells: Mechanical Properties, Cell Viability, and Function. *Biomacromolecules* **2003**, *4*, 890–895. [CrossRef]
48. Van Wachem, P.B.; Plantinga, J.A.; Wissink, M.J.B.; Beernink, R.; Poot, A.A.; Engbers, G.H.M.; Beugeling, T.; Van Aken, W.G.; Feijen, J.; Van Luyn, M.J.A. In Vivo biocompatibility of carbodiimide-crosslinked collagen matrices: Effects of crosslink density, heparin immobilization, and bFGF loading. *J. Biomed. Mater. Res.* **2001**, *55*, 368–378. [CrossRef]
49. Alessandrino, A.; Chiarini, A.; Biagiotti, M.; Dal Prà, I.; Bassani, G.A.; Vincoli, V.; Settembrini, P.; Pierimarchi, P.; Freddi, G.; Armato, U. Three-Layered Silk Fibroin Tubular Scaold for the Repair and Regeneration of Small Caliber Blood Vessels: From Design to in vivo Pilot Tests. *Front. Bioeng. Biotechnol.* **2019**, *7*, 356. [CrossRef]
50. Asakura, T.; Tanaka, T.; Tanaka, R. Advanced Silk Fibroin Biomaterials and Application to Small-Diameter Silk Vascular Grafts. *ACS Biomater. Sci. Eng.* **2018**, *5*, 5561–5577. [CrossRef]
51. Rockwood, D.N.; Preda, R.C.; Yücel, T.; Wang, X.; Lovett, M.L.; Kaplan, D.L. Materials fabrication from Bombyx mori silk fibroin. *Nat. Protoc.* **2011**, *6*, 1612–1631. [CrossRef] [PubMed]
52. Teuschl, A.H.; Van Griensven, M.; Redl, H. Sericin Removal from Raw Bombyx mori Silk Scaffolds of High Hierarchical Order. *Tissue Eng. Part C Methods* **2014**, *20*, 431–439. [CrossRef]
53. Kunz, R.I.; Brancalhão, R.M.C.; Ribeiro, L.D.F.C.; Natali, M.R.M. Silkworm Sericin: Properties and Biomedical Applications. *BioMed Res. Int.* **2016**, *2016*, 1–19. [CrossRef]
54. Puerta, M.; Montoya, Y.; Bustamante, J.; Restrepo-Osorio, A. Potential Applications of Silk Fibroin as Vascular Implants: A Review. *Crit. Rev. Biomed. Eng.* **2019**, *47*, 365–378. [CrossRef] [PubMed]
55. Enomoto, S.; Sumi, M.; Kajimoto, K.; Nakazawa, Y.; Takahashi, R.; Takabayashi, C.; Asakura, T.; Sata, M. Long-Term patency of small-diameter vascular graft made from fibroin, a silk-based biodegradable material. *J. Vasc. Surg.* **2010**, *51*, 155–164. [CrossRef]
56. Aper, T.; Teebken, O.; Steinhoff, G.; Haverich, A. Use of a Fibrin Preparation in the Engineering of a Vascular Graft Model. *Eur. J. Vasc. Endovasc. Surg.* **2004**, *28*, 296–302. [CrossRef]
57. Weisel, J.W.; Litvinov, R.I. Fibrin Formation, Structure and Properties. *Subcell. Biochem.* **2017**, *82*, 405–456.
58. Zhu, M.; Li, W.; Dong, X.; Yuan, X.; Midgley, A.; Chang, H.; Wang, Y.; Wang, H.; Wang, K.; Ma, P.X.; et al. In Vivo engineered extracellular matrix scaffolds with instructive niches for oriented tissue regeneration. *Nat. Commun.* **2019**, *10*, 1–14. [CrossRef]
59. Smith, R.J., Jr.; Nasiri, B.; Kann, J.; Yergeau, D.; Bard, J.E.; Swartz, D.D.; Andreadis, S.T. Endothelialization of arterial vascular grafts by circulating monocytes. *Nat. Commun.* **2020**, *11*, 1622. [CrossRef]
60. Arasu, R.; Campbell, I.; Cartmill, A.; Cohen, T.; Hansen, P.; Muller, J.; Dave, R.; McGahan, T. Management of primary mycotic aneurysms and prosthetic graft infections: An 8-year experience with in-situ cryopreserved allograft reconstruction. *ANZ J. Surg.* **2020**, *90*, 1716–1720. [CrossRef] [PubMed]
61. Stanislawski, N.; Cholewa, F.; Heymann, H.; Kraus, X.; Heene, S.; Witt, M.; Thoms, S.; Blume, C.; Blume, H. Automated Bioreactor System for the Cultivation of Autologous Tissue-Engineered Vascular Grafts. *Annu. Int. Conf. IEEE Eng. Med. Biol. Soc.* **2020**, *2020*, 2257–2261. [CrossRef] [PubMed]

62. Mallis, P.; Michalopoulos, E.; Pantsios, P.; Kozaniti, F.; Deligianni, D.; Papapanagiotou, A.; Giokas, C.S. Recellularization potential of small diameter vascular grafts derived from human umbilical artery. *Bio. Med. Mater. Eng.* **2019**, *30*, 61–71. [CrossRef]
63. Hillebrandt, K.H.; Everwien, H.; Haep, N.; Keshi, E.; Pratschke, J.; Sauer, I. Strategies based on organ decellularization and recellularization. *Transpl. Int.* **2019**, *32*, 571–585. [CrossRef] [PubMed]
64. Badylak, S.F.; Taylor, D.; Uygun, K. Whole-Organ Tissue Engineering: Decellularization and Recellularization of Three-Dimensional Matrix Scaffolds. *Annu. Rev. Biomed. Eng.* **2011**, *13*, 27–53. [CrossRef] [PubMed]
65. Tuschong, L.; Soenen, S.L.; Blaese, R.M.; Candotti, F.; Muul, L.M. Immune response to foetal calf serum by two adenosine deaminase-deficient patients after T cell gene therapy. *Hum. Gene Ther.* **2002**, *13*, 1605–1610. [CrossRef] [PubMed]
66. Jung, S.; Panchalingam, K.; Rosenberg, L.; Behie, L.A. Ex VivoExpansion of Human Mesenchymal Stem Cells in Defined Serum-Free Media. *Stem Cells Int.* **2012**, *2012*, 1–21. [CrossRef]
67. Schallmoser, K.; Bartmann, C.; Rohde, E.; Reinisch, A.; Kashofer, K.; Stadelmeyer, E.; Drexler, C.; Lanzer, G.; Linkesch, W.; Strunk, D. Human platelet lysate can replace foetal bovine serum for clinical-scale expansion of functional mesenchymal stromal cells. *Transfusion* **2007**, *47*, 1436–1446. [CrossRef]
68. Bieback, K.; Hecker, A.; Kocaomer, A.; Lannert, H.; Schallmoser, K.; Strunk, D.; Ter, H. Human alternatives to foetal bovine serum for the expansion of mesenchymal stromal cells from bone marrow. *Stem Cells* **2009**, *27*, 2331–2341. [CrossRef]
69. Mallis, P.; Alevrogianni, V.; Sarri, P.; Velentzas, A.D.; Stavropoulos-Giokas, C.; Michalopoulos, E. Effect of Cord Blood Platelet Gel on wound healing capacity of human Mesenchymal Stromal Cells. *Transfus. Apher. Sci.* **2020**, *59*, 102734. [CrossRef]
70. Mallis, P.; Papapanagiotou, A.; Katsimpoulas, M.; Kostakis, A.; Siasos, G.; Kassi, E.; Stavropoulos-Giokas, C.; Michalopoulos, E. Efficient differentiation of vascular smooth muscle cells from Wharton's Jelly mesenchymal stromal cells using human platelet lysate: A potential cell source for small blood vessel engineering. *World J. Stem Cells* **2020**, *12*, 203–221. [CrossRef]
71. Bellis, S.L. Advantages of RGD peptides for directing cell association with biomaterials. *Biomaterials* **2011**, *32*, 4205–4210. [CrossRef]
72. Huebsch, J.C.; McCarthy, J.B.; Diglio, C.A.; Mooradian, D.L. Endothelial Cell Interactions With Synthetic Peptides From the Carboxyl-Terminal Heparin-Binding Domains of Fibronectin. *Circ. Res.* **1995**, *77*, 43–53. [CrossRef]
73. Mallis, P.; Sokolis, D.P.; Makridakis, M.; Zoidakis, J.; Velentzas, A.D.; Katsimpoulas, M.; Vlahou, A.; Kostakis, A.; Stavropoulos-Giokas, C.; Michalopoulos, E. Insights into Biomechanical and Proteomic Characteristics of Small Diameter Vascular Grafts Utilizing the Human Umbilical Artery. *Biomedicines* **2020**, *8*, 280. [CrossRef]
74. Dimitrievska, S.; Cai, C.; Weyers, A.; Balestrini, J.L.; Lin, T.; Sundaram, S.; Hatachi, G.; Spiegel, D.A.; Kyriakides, T.R.; Miao, J.; et al. Click-Coated, heparinized, decellularized vascular grafts. *Acta Biomater.* **2015**, *13*, 177–187. [CrossRef]
75. Koobatian, M.T.; Row, S.; Smith, R.J., Jr.; Koenigsknecht, C.; Andreadis, S.T.; Swartz, D.D. Successful endothelialization and remodeling of a cell-free small-diameter arterial graft in a large animal model. *Biomaterials* **2015**, *76*, 344–358. [CrossRef] [PubMed]
76. Sexton, A.J.; Turmaine, M.; Cai, W.Q.; Burnstock, G. A study of the ultrastructure of developing human umbilical vessels. *J. Anat.* **1996**, *188*, 75–85.
77. Roy, S.; Silacci, P.; Stergiopulos, N. Biomechanical properties of decellularized porcine common carotid arteries. *Am. J. Physiol. Heart Circ. Physiol.* **2005**, *289*, H1567–H1576. [CrossRef]
78. Marino, L.; Castaldi, M.A.; Rosamilio, R.; Ragni, E.; Vitolo, R.; Fulgione, C.; Castaldi, S.G.; Serio, B.; Bianco, R.; Guida, M.; et al. Mesenchymal Stem Cells from the Wharton's Jelly of the Human Umbilical Cord: Biological Properties and Therapeutic Potential. *Int. J. Stem Cells* **2019**, *12*, 218–226. [CrossRef]
79. Mallis, P.; Michalopoulos, E.; Chatzistamatiou, T.; Stavropoulos-Giokas, C. Mesenchymal stromal cells as potential immunomodulatory players in severe acute respiratory distress syndrome induced by SARS-CoV-2 infection. *World J. Stem Cells* **2020**, *12*, 731–751. [CrossRef] [PubMed]
80. Mallis, P.; Michalopoulos, E.; Chatzistamatiou, T.; Giokas, C.S. Interplay between mesenchymal stromal cells and immune system: Clinical applications in immune-related diseases. *Explor. Immunol.* **2021**, *1*, 112–139. [CrossRef]
81. Via, A.G.; Frizziero, A.; Oliva, F. Biological properties of mesenchymal Stem Cells from different sources. *Muscle Ligaments Tendons J.* **2012**, *2*, 154–162.
82. Chen, J.-Y.; Mou, X.-Z.; Du, X.-C.; Xiang, C. Comparative analysis of biological characteristics of adult mesenchymal stem cells with different tissue origins. *Asian Pac. J. Trop. Med.* **2015**, *8*, 739–746. [CrossRef]
83. Stewart, M.C.; Stewart, A.A. Mesenchymal stem cells: Characteristics, sources, and mechanisms of action. *Vet. Clin. N. Am. Equine Pract.* **2011**, *27*, 243–261. [CrossRef]
84. Doucet, C.; Ernou, I.; Zhang, Y.; Llense, J.-R.; Begot, L.; Holy, X.; Lataillade, J.-J. Platelet lysates promote mesenchymal stem cell expansion: A safety substitute for animal serum in cell-based therapy applications. *J. Cell. Physiol.* **2005**, *205*, 228–236. [CrossRef] [PubMed]
85. Jooybar, E.; Abdekhodaie, M.J.; Alvi, M.; Mousavi, A.; Karperien, M.; Dijkstra, P.J. An injectable platelet lysate-hyaluronic acid hydrogel supports cellular activities and induces chondrogenesis of encapsulated mesenchymal stem cells. *Acta Biomater.* **2018**, *83*, 233–244. [CrossRef] [PubMed]
86. Zhang, L.; Qiu, H.; Wang, D.; Miao, H.; Zhu, Y.; Guo, Q.; Guo, Y.; Wang, Z. Enhanced vascularization and biocompatibility of rat pancreatic decellularized scaffolds loaded with platelet-rich plasma. *J. Biomater. Appl.* **2020**, *35*, 313–330. [CrossRef]
87. Mebratu, Y.; Tesfaigzi, Y. How ERK1/2 activation controls cell proliferation and cell death: Is subcellular localization the answer? *Cell Cycle* **2009**, *8*, 1168–1175. [CrossRef] [PubMed]

88. Lee, J.G.; Kay, E.P. PI 3-kinase/Rac1 and ERK1/2 regulate FGF-2-mediated cell proliferation through phosphorylation of p27 at Ser10 by KIS and at Thr187 by Cdc25A/Cdk2. *Invest Ophthalmol. Vis. Sci.* **2011**, *52*, 417–426. [CrossRef]
89. Lefloch, R.; Pouysségur, J.; Lenormand, P. Total ERK1/2 activity regulates cell proliferation. *Cell Cycle* **2009**, *8*, 705–711. [CrossRef] [PubMed]
90. Meloche, S.; Pouysségur, J. The ERK1/2 mitogen-activated protein kinase pathway as a master regulator of the G1- to S-phase transition. *Oncogene* **2007**, *26*, 3227–3239. [CrossRef]
91. Servant, M.J.; Giasson, E.; Meloche, S. Inhibition of Growth Factor-induced Protein Synthesis by a Selective MEK Inhibitor in Aortic Smooth Muscle Cells. *J. Biol. Chem.* **1996**, *271*, 16047–16052. [CrossRef]
92. Treinies, I.; Paterson, H.F.; Hooper, S.; Wilson, R.; Marshall, C.J. Activated MEK Stimulates Expression of AP-1 Components Independently of Phosphatidylinositol 3-Kinase (PI3-Kinase) but Requires a PI3-Kinase Signal To Stimulate DNA Synthesis. *Mol. Cell. Biol.* **1999**, *19*, 321–329. [CrossRef]
93. Gotoh, I.; Fukuda, M.; Adachi, M.; Nishida, E. Control of the Cell Morphology and the S Phase Entry by Mitogen-activated Protein Kinase Kinase: A Regulatory Role of Its N-Terminal Region. *J. Biol. Chem.* **1999**, *274*, 11874–11880. [CrossRef] [PubMed]
94. Force, T.; Bonventre, J.V. Growth Factors and Mitogen-Activated Protein Kinases. *Hypertension* **1998**, *31*, 152–161. [CrossRef] [PubMed]
95. Katz, M.; Amit, I.; Yarden, Y. Regulation of MAPKs by growth factors and receptor tyrosine kinases. *Biochim. Biophys. Acta Bioenerg.* **2007**, *1773*, 1161–1176. [CrossRef]
96. Page, K.; Li, J.; Hershenson, M.B. Platelet-Derived Growth Factor Stimulation of Mitogen-Activated Protein Kinases and Cyclin D1Promoter Activity in Cultured Airway Smooth-Muscle Cells. *Am. J. Respir. Cell Mol. Biol.* **1999**, *20*, 1294–1302. [CrossRef]
97. Yang, Q.E.; Giassetti, M.I.; Ealy, A.D. Fibroblast growth factors activate mitogen-activated protein kinase pathways to promote migration in ovine trophoblast cells. *Reproduction* **2011**, *141*, 707–714. [CrossRef]

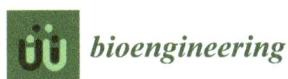

Article

Biomimetic 3D Models for Investigating the Role of Monocytes and Macrophages in Atherosclerosis

Anna Garcia-Sabaté [1], Walaa Kamal E. Mohamed [1,2], Jiranuwat Sapudom [1], Aseel Alatoom [1], Layla Al Safadi [1] and Jeremy C. M. Teo [1,3,*]

1. Laboratory for Immuno Bioengineering Research and Applications, Division of Engineering, New York University Abu Dhabi, 129188 Abu Dhabi, UAE; anna.sabate@nyu.edu (A.G.-S.); wm1081@nyu.edu (W.K.E.M.); jiranuwat.sapudom@nyu.edu (J.S.); aseel.alatoom@nyu.edu (A.A.); las892@nyu.edu (L.A.S.)
2. Departament de Genètica i Microbiologia, Facultat de Biociències, Universitat Autònoma de Bellaterra, 08193 Barcelona, Spain
3. Department of Mechanical and Biomedical Engineering, Tandon School of Engineering, New York University, New York, NY 11201, USA
* Correspondence: jeremy.teo@nyu.edu; Tel.: +971-2-628-6689

Received: 25 August 2020; Accepted: 14 September 2020; Published: 16 September 2020

Abstract: Atherosclerosis, the inflammation of artery walls due to the accumulation of lipids, is the most common underlying cause for cardiovascular diseases. Monocytes and macrophages are major cells that contribute to the initiation and progression of atherosclerotic plaques. During this process, an accumulation of LDL-laden macrophages (foam cells) and an alteration in the extracellular matrix (ECM) organization leads to a local vessel stiffening. Current in vitro models are carried out onto two-dimensional tissue culture plastic and cannot replicate the relevant microenvironments. To bridge the gap between in vitro and in vivo conditions, we utilized three-dimensional (3D) collagen matrices that allowed us to mimic the ECM stiffening during atherosclerosis by increasing collagen density. First, human monocytic THP-1 cells were embedded into 3D collagen matrices reconstituted at low and high density. Cells were subsequently differentiated into uncommitted macrophages (M0) and further activated into pro- (M1) and anti-inflammatory (M2) phenotypes. In order to mimic atherosclerotic conditions, cells were cultured in the presence of oxidized LDL (oxLDL) and analyzed in terms of oxLDL uptake capability and relevant receptors along with their cytokine secretomes. Although oxLDL uptake and larger lipid size could be observed in macrophages in a matrix dependent manner, monocytes showed higher numbers of oxLDL uptake cells. By analyzing major oxLDL uptake receptors, both monocytes and macrophages expressed lectin-like oxidized low-density lipoprotein receptor-1 (LOX1), while enhanced expression of scavenger receptor CD36 could be observed only in M2. Notably, by analyzing the secretome of macrophages exposed to oxLDL, we demonstrated that the cells could, in fact, secrete adipokines and growth factors in distinct patterns. Besides, oxLDL appeared to up-regulate MHCII expression in all cells, while an up-regulation of CD68, a pan-macrophage marker, was found only in monocytes, suggesting a possible differentiation of monocytes into a pro-inflammatory macrophage. Overall, our work demonstrated that collagen density in the plaque could be one of the major factors driving atherosclerotic progression via modulation of monocyte and macrophages behaviors.

Keywords: atherosclerosis; monocyte; macrophage; disease model; collagen; 3D cell culture; immunomechanobiology

1. Introduction

Atherosclerosis is the dominant underlying causation of coronary heart disease and cerebrovascular disease [1] and statistically a major cause of morbidity and mortality worldwide [2,3]. The systematic formation of detrimental atherosclerotic plaques, via monocyte to macrophage differentiation to foam cell formation, which eventually narrows and occludes arteries, is well-reviewed elsewhere [4,5]. In short, monocytes are recruited to lesion sites, where low-density lipoproteins (LDL) and apolipoprotein B-containing lipoproteins have accumulated and activated the endothelium. Monocytes then infiltrate the lesion and differentiate into macrophages, which will uptake lipoproteins, ultimately resulting in foam cells that comprise the central core of atheromas that will progressively occlude the vessel. Atherosclerosis is considered a non-resolving inflammatory condition [2,6], akin to chronic wounds that will not resolve towards healing. On account of this close association with wound healing, and evidence that atherosclerotic plaques are vastly populated by pan-macrophage marker CD68+ cells, macrophages are thought to play other lead roles beyond foam cell formation that progresses plaque buildup [7,8].

In atherosclerosis, macrophages are implicated in progression or regression of plaques, as well as in plaque stabilization or its rupture [9,10]. Pro-inflammatory macrophages, or M1 macrophages, are responsible for progression, leading towards instability and finally resulting in rupture [11]. Conventionally, at the complete opposite end of the macrophage spectrum, sits the anti-inflammatory or M2 macrophages [12], which mediate a more favorable outcome of atherosclerosis [13]. It is now accepted that macrophage phenotypes are not dichotomous but lie along this M1-M2 spectrum, and depending on the atherosclerotic cellular niche, macrophages can dynamically traverse this M1-M2 continuum [12,14], affecting the outcome of this disease. While significant advancements have been made in terms of disease management, research must now shift towards understanding the mechanisms of atherosclerosis regression and the repair of atherosclerotic lesions [15]. It is, therefore, imperative to understand macrophage biology in the interest of this new pivot against atherosclerosis.

Animal models have provided abundant information for atherosclerosis research, however, to understand atherosclerosis healing mechanistically, relevant in vitro models are a must. Models of atherosclerosis have progressed from simple 2D culture to 3D multi-cellular cultures [16,17], the latter a better representation considering the dimensionality of the disease and anatomical features involved. To mimic in vivo-like conditions, in vitro models have encapsulated the relevant cells of interest within naturally-derived and polymer-based hydrogels.

Several 3D models of atherosclerosis have been published [18–21]. While they mostly tackled the interaction between different cells in atherosclerotic plaques at different stages of plaque progression, they overlooked some factors which we aim to address. The 3D extracellular matrix (ECM) used for scaffolding the models was not assessed in terms of its biomechanical influence on monocytes and macrophages in regard to atherosclerosis' cellular niche. This is especially important since collagen comprises up to 60% of the plaque protein [22], and the amount of collagen in the plaque dictates its mechanical stability [23], where a deficiency of collagen may lead to plaque rupture and an excess results in narrowing of the artery. Moreover, aged or obese individuals are known to exhibit notably stiffened and thickened arteries [24]. Also, our previous work has specifically shown that macrophage functionality and immune phenotype is regulated by physical parameters of the surrounding ECM [25]. While the majority of biological readouts from 2D and 3D in vitro atherosclerosis models have focused on LDL uptake by the immune cells and secretion of specific pro-inflammatory cytokines, there is a lack of comprehensive secretome studies. Owing to the complexity of the biochemical milieu in atherosclerotic microenvironments, we want to examine adipokines and growth factors, two groups of cytokines that are currently vague, but crucial to understanding the mechanisms of regression and repair of atherosclerotic plaques. Furthermore, most 3D models commonly employ monocytes or resident macrophages (M0) for LDL exposure to simulate atherosclerosis. However, there are pathological situations, for example, dyslipidemia, diabetes, hypertension, obesity, and smoking, whereby transendothelial permeability to LDLs increases [26,27] and resident macrophages of varying phenotypes within the intima could uptake LDLs, thus also modulate atherosclerotic plaque [14].

In this study, we employ a system of collagen-based hydrogels with different matrix densities that recapitulate the porosity of early (low tissue density) and advanced (high tissue density) atherosclerotic tissue in vivo [28,29]. Within these fibrillar collagen hydrogels, a commonly used and genetically uniform human monocytic cell line, THP-1, is embedded, differentiated into various macrophage phenotypes, and later exposed to oxidized LDLs (oxLDL). Here, we aim to elucidate the effects of the predominant ECM, collagen, on these immune cells by isolating them from other factors such as different cell types or proteins. The assessment was performed to evaluate oxLDL uptake, scavenger receptors and immune phenotype gene expressions, and their secretions of adipokine and growth factors.

2. Materials and Methods

2.1. Cell Culture

Human monocytic cell line THP-1 were maintained in RPMI-1640 (Gibco, Thermo Fisher Scientific, Inc., Waltham, MA, USA) with 10% fetal bovine serum (FBS), 1% HEPES, 1% sodium pyruvate, 0.01% beta-mercaptoethanol, and 1% penicillin/streptomycin (all from Invitrogen, Thermo Fisher Scientific, Inc.) at 37 °C, 95% humidity and 5% CO_2 (standard cell culture conditions).

2.2. Embedding and Differentiating THP-1 towards Macrophages in 3D Collagen Matrices

3D collagen matrices at concentrations of 1 and 3 mg/mL were prepared as previously published [25,30]. In short, a collagen solution was prepared by mixing of type I rat tail collagen (Advanced BioMatrix, Inc., Carlsbad, CA, USA) with 250 mM of phosphate buffer and 0.1% acetic acid (both from Sigma-Aldrich, Inc., St. Louis, MO, USA). Afterward, 1×10^5 THP-1 cells were suspended in the prepared collagen solution and then transferred onto glutaraldehyde-coated coverslips. Cell-free collagen matrices were analyzed prior to use for cell culture regarding their topological and mechanical properties, using an image-based analysis toolbox [31] and non-destructive rheometer [25,32], respectively.

Macrophage differentiation was performed using an established protocol [25]. In brief, THP-1 cells were differentiated into uncommitted macrophages (M0) by culturing in RPMI 1640 media without FBS supplemented with 300 nM phorbol 12-myristate 13-acetate (PMA; Sigma-Aldrich, Inc.) for 6 h. To achieve pro-inflammatory (M1) and anti-inflammatory (M2) macrophages, PMA containing media was removed, and M0 were rested in RPMI-1640 cell culture media without FBS for 24 h. Afterward, cells were cultured in activating media for 48 h. For M1 activation, RPMI-1640 cell culture media without FBS was supplemented with 10 pg/mL lipopolysaccharide (LPS, Sigma-Aldrich, Inc.) and 20 ng/mL interferon-gamma IFN-γ (Biolegend, Inc., San Diego, CA, USA), while 20 ng/mL interleukin 4 (IL-4, Biolegend, Inc.) and 20 ng/mL interleukin 13 (IL-13, Biolegend, Inc.) was used for M2 activation.

2.3. Topological and Mechanical Characterization of 3D Collagen Matrices

Cell-free 3D collagen matrices were analyzed regarding their topological and mechanical properties based on previously published protocols [32]. In brief, 5- (and-6)-carboxytetramethylrhodaminesuccinimidylester (5(6)-TAMRA-SE) (Sigma-Aldrich, Inc.) stained 3D collagen matrices were imaged using confocal microscopy (SP8; Leica Microsystems GmbH, Wetzlar, Germany) at 63X. Z-stacked (50 μm depth, at 5 μm intervals) image datasets (of pixel size 0.13×0.13 μm) were analyzed using a custom-built image analysis toolbox [31] to obtain mean pore size. For each type of 3D collagen matrix, analysis was performed in triplicate with three positions per sample. Measurements of mechanical properties was performed on cell-free label-free 3D collagen matrices non-destructively (ElastoSense™ Bio; Rheolution Inc., Montreal, QC, Canada).

Briefly, fibrillation of 3 mL of collagen solution was initiated at 37 °C and the elastic modulus of collagen was measured during polymerization. Three samples per matrix type were analyzed.

2.4. Treatment with oxLDL

Monocyte (THP-1), plus uncommitted and activated macrophages were cultured in the presence of 5 µg/mL oxidized low-density lipoproteins from human plasma (oxLDL; Molecular Probes™, Thermo Fisher Scientific, Inc.) for 5 days at standard cell culture condition. oxLDL conjugated 1,1′-dioctadecyl-3,3,3′,3′-tetramethylindocarbocyanine perchlorate (DiI) was used for quantification and visualization of LDL uptake. As a control, cells were cultured at similar conditions without oxLDL.

2.5. Quantitative Analysis of oxLDL Uptake

After 5 days of LDL treatment, collagen matrices were digested with 6 mg/mL of collagenase (Worthington Biochemical Corp., Lakewood, NJ, USA) prepared in cell culture media for 15 min at standard cell culture conditions to digest the collagen. Afterward, cells were analyzed using Attune NxT Flow Cytometer equipped with autosampler (Thermo Fisher Scientific, Inc.). Percentage of oxLDL uptake cells and mean fluorescent intensity were quantified using FlowJow Software (Build 10.5.3; BD Life Sciences). Experiments were performed in 5 replicates.

2.6. Quantitative Analysis of Lipid Droplet Size

For analysis of lipid droplet size, cells were first fixed with 4% paraformaldehyde and stained with 4′,6-diamidino-2-phenylindole (DAPI; 1:10,000 dilution in PBS) for 2 h at room temperature. Afterward, cells were imaged using a confocal laser scanning microscope (cLSM) (SP8; Leica Microsystems GmbH). The cLSM stacked images were gathered and analyzed regarding the lipid size using DiI-oxLDL fluorescence signal by a home-built MATLAB script (MATLAB 2019a; The MathWorks, Inc., Natick, MA, USA).

2.7. Quantitative Analysis of Adipokines, Chemoattractants, and Growth Factors

Secretion of adipokines, chemoattractants, and growth factors were analyzed from cell culture supernatant after 5 days of cell culture in the presence and absence of oxLDL. Custom bead-based multiplex immunoassays were used to quantify secretome (Biolegend, Inc.), following the manufacturer's instructions. Samples were analyzed using Attune NxT Flow Cytometer equipped with autosampler (Thermo Fisher Scientific, Inc.). Data analysis was done using LEGENDplex™ Data Analysis Software (Biolegend, Inc.).

2.8. Gene Expression Analysis

Gene expression analysis was performed using an established protocol, as published [25]. Briefly, total RNA was extracted using TRIzol (Invitrogen, Thermo Fisher Scientific, Inc.) and converted into complementary DNA (cDNA) using a high-capacity cDNA reverse transcription kit (Applied Biosystems, Thermo Fisher Scientific, Inc.). The cDNA concentration and purity (the ratio of absorbance at 260 nm and 280 nm) were quantified using nanodrops (Thermo Fisher Scientific, Inc.) prior to performing gene expression analysis. The primers used in this study were synthesized from Bioneer Inc. The primer sequences are listed in Supplementary Table S1. qPCR was performed using the SYBR Green PCR Master Mix (Applied Biosystems, Thermo Fisher Scientific, Inc.). The qPCR procedure was set as follows: denaturation for 5 min at 95 °C; 45 cycles of denaturation (95 °C, 15 s), annealing under primer-specific conditions (30 s), and target gene-specific extension (30 s at 72 °C). Fluorescence signals were measured for 20 s at 72 °C. To confirm the specificity of the PCR products, a melting curve analysis was performed at the end of each run. The Beta-actin gene was used as a reference gene. Experiments were performed in four replicates.

2.9. Data and Statistical Analysis

Unless otherwise stated, all experiments were performed in at least four repeats, and data are represented as mean ± standard deviation (SD). Statistical significance has been determined by two-way ANOVA followed by Tukey's test using Prism 8 (GraphPad Software), and the level of significance was set to $p < 0.05$, unless otherwise stated.

3. Results

With atherosclerosis being the main cause of cardiovascular diseases [1], there is an increasing need for platforms that can mimic in vivo conditions. Furthermore, these platforms must be thoroughly characterized, and a profound understanding of individual contributions of the cells involved in atherosclerosis development must be reached before venturing to co-culture models. Most atherosclerosis studies are carried on 2D tissue culture plates [16]. While meaningful contributions have been made towards 3D modeling atherosclerosis in vitro, most studies have focused on co-culture of endothelial cells (ECs), smooth muscle cells (SMCs), and monocytes, in either physiological [18] or synthetic [20] scaffolds, while detailed individual contributions of macrophages still remain unclear.

Here, we embedded monocytic THP-1 cells into 3D type I collagen matrices of low and high concentrations, surrogates for the plaque of low and high densities. As mentioned earlier, collagen I is known to make up for approximately two-thirds of the total collagen in atherosclerotic plaques [22], and the progression of atherosclerosis leads to an increase in collagen concentration within the different layers of diseased vessels. By reconstituting collagen matrices at low and high densities, we were able to mimic the changes of the ECM at early and advanced stages of atherosclerosis. The pore size of the collagen matrices was 11.54 ± 0.88 µm and 3.67 ± 0.95 µm for 1 mg/mL and 3 mg/mL collagen concentration, respectively, and as expected, matrix elasticity was enhanced with an increase of collagen concentration and was 52.10 ± 10.38 Pa and 211.43 ± 15.62 Pa for 1 mg/mL and 3 mg/mL collagen concentration, respectively. The resulting pore sizes span the pore sizes found in vivo [28,30]. Those of atherosclerotic plaque have not been experimentally measured as far as we know, likely due to the complexity of such tissues. However, it has been reported that regressive plaques (i.e., more advanced) have an increased content of collagen [33]. Embedded cells were differentiated into macrophages and further activated into distinct pro- and anti-inflammatory phenotypes. Cells were cultured in the presence of oxLDL simulating atherosclerosis conditions in vitro for 5 days. The duration of the treatment was experimentally determined by measuring oxLDL uptake at different timepoints, we observed that engulfment of LDL by all cells plateaued from 5 days onwards (data not shown). To understand the differences in response by each cell type, we evaluate the uptake of lipids, further assess their expression of relevant oxLDL receptors, quantified their secretomes, and finally examined their expression of selected surface markers to discern if there are any phenotypic changes due to oxLDL exposure.

3.1. %oxLDL + Cells Are Greatest in Monocytes and M1 Accumulates the Most oxLDL

Monocytes and macrophages were cultured in the presence and absence of DiI fluorescent-tagged oxLDL (DiI-oxLDL) for 5 days. As shown in Figure 1A, it can be observed that macrophages uptake a higher amount of oxLDL than monocytes, and particularly M1 appears to engulf more oxLDL than other macrophage phenotypes. No differences in uptake could be visually observed between low and high matrix density for the same cell phenotypes. To confirm the visual impressions, cells were harvested from 3D collagen matrices by digestion with collagenase and oxLDL uptake was analyzed by flow cytometry. The percentage of oxLDL positive cells (oxLDL+ cells; cells that uptake oxLDL) and the uptake capacity were assessed using mean fluorescence intensity (MFI). As shown in Figure 1B, we observed a significantly high percentage of monocytes that uptake oxLDL when compared to macrophages (see Supplementary Figure S1A). However, monocytes engulf a lower amount of oxLDL, as demonstrated through MFI. M1 showed significantly higher uptake compared to M0 and M2 macrophages (Supplementary Figure S1B) but without significant difference across matrix densities. We further quantified the size of lipid droplets using a custom-built image analysis toolbox written in MATLAB. Interestingly, we found larger lipid droplets in low matrix density in all macrophage phenotypes, while no differences could be observed in monocytes.

In sum, our results suggest higher oxLDL uptake in all macrophages, especially in M1 phenotypes, than in monocytes. This finding is in line with the high phagocytic activity of M1 macrophages [34], while it contradicts reports that showed M2 macrophages have a higher capacity to accumulate LDL than M1 in the 2D culture model [35,36]. Literature reports that M1 macrophages are the predominant phenotype present in human and mouse plaque lesions and directly contribute to atherosclerotic plaque formation in vivo [11,37–40], which supports our findings in the 3D cell culture model. Both %oxLDL+ cells, as well as lipid size, was reduced in higher density matrices.

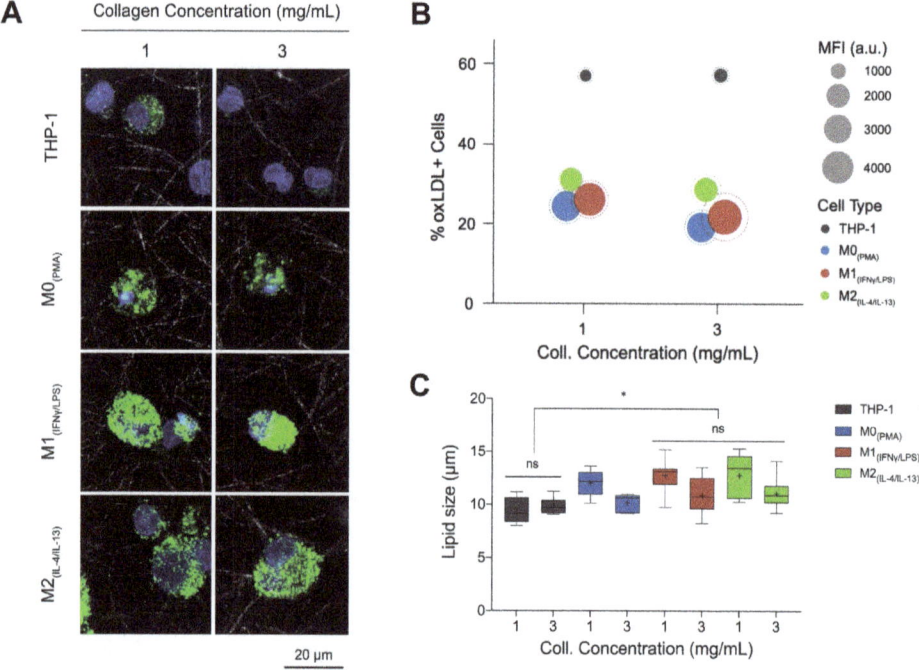

Figure 1. oxLDL uptake by monocytes and macrophages in 3D collagen matrices. (**A**) Representative confocal images of monocytes and macrophages with DiI-oxLDL uptake. (**B**) In this infographic, the number of oxLDL+ cells (y-axis) was greatest in THP-1 (grey) followed by M2 (green) macrophages, then M1 (red), and finally M0 (blue). The amount of oxLDL in the cells, as quantified through mean fluorescence intensity (MFI, solid circle) (circle size, see legend), was greatest in M1 macrophages, followed by M0, then M2, and finally THP-1. The dotted circle is the corresponding standard deviation of the MFI. A sample size of 5 was performed for each condition. (**C**) Lipid droplet size as measured from images obtained with confocal microscopy using a custom-built image analysis toolbox. Data were shown as a boxplot (whiskers represent minimum and maximum, + represents the mean, line inside each box plot represents the median). Significance is represented as * $p < 0.05$ between samples in 1 mg/mL collagen concentration.

3.2. oxLDL Induced LOX1 Expression in Monocytes and Macrophages, while It Enhanced CD36 Expression in M2 Phenotypes

To better understand the oxLDL uptake and lipid size formation, we assessed if the presence of oxLDL affects its uptake receptors. We analyzed the gene expression profile of two main receptors responsible for oxLDL uptake, namely lectin-like oxidized low-density lipoprotein receptor-1 (*LOX1*) and scavenger receptor class B member 3 (*CD36*) through qPCR [41,42]. LOX1 is a transmembrane glycoprotein that binds to and internalizes oxLDL resulting in distinct cell-type-specific downstream signaling, which leads to differential cellular behaviors [43]. As shown in Figure 2A, in the absence of oxLDL, no significant change in LOX1 could be observed between monocytes and macrophages as well as between matrix density. After treatment with oxLDL, all cells exhibited up-regulation of LOX1 expression with the highest expression in M1, tying in with our MFI data, followed by M2, M0 macrophages, and then monocytes. Our finding is corroborated by other reports suggesting an enhanced LOX1 expression via activated nuclear factor kappa-light-chain-enhancer of activated B cells (NF-kB) [44], pro-inflammatory cytokines mediated LOX1 expression [45], as well as oxidative stress [46]. The mentioned mechanisms might also explain the higher expression of LOX1 in M1 phenotypes. Contradicting our MFI data, we found slightly higher expression in the dense matrix in monocytes and macrophages, except M2 phenotypes. We postulate that this observation might be caused by an enhanced modulation of pro-inflammatory response by macrophages in a dense matrix, as previously reported [25]. Further evidence that collagen concentration can modulate the phenotype of macrophages is found in atherosclerotic plaque progression and regression studies [47–49], where progressive plaques (lower collagen content) contain more pro-inflammatory macrophages, while more anti-inflammatory macrophages are found in regressive plaques (higher collagen content).

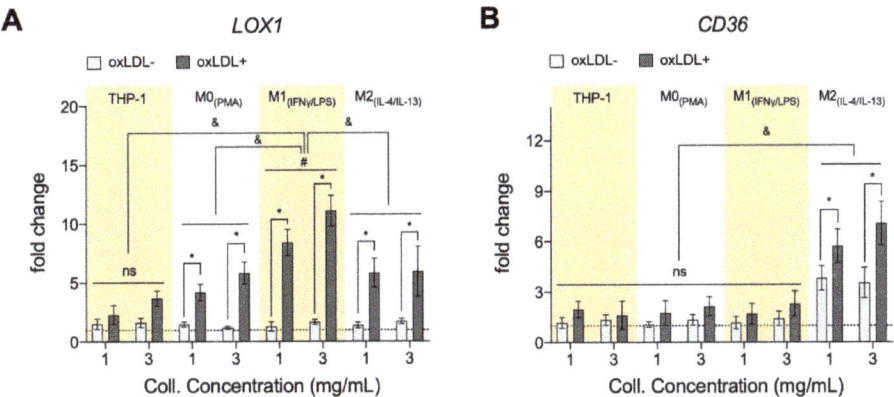

Figure 2. Expression of oxLDL receptors of monocytes and macrophages cultured in 3D collagen matrices. (**A**) There is an increase in gene expression of lectin-like oxidized low-density lipoprotein receptor-1 (*LOX1*) in both monocytes (THP-1) and significantly in all macrophage subtypes when cells are cultured in 3D collagen hydrogels and exposed to oxLDL. Significantly, M1$_{+LDL}$ exhibited the highest fold induction and THP-1$_{+LDL}$, the lowest, with M0$_{+LDL}$ and M2$_{+LDL}$ comparable. LOX1 expression only changed significantly in M1 with collagen concentration (x-axis, 1 mg/mL to 3 mg/mL). (**B**) Genetic expression of *CD36*, another oxLDL receptor, was only measurable in M2$_{+LDL}$, and significantly higher expression was found in lower density collagen hydrogels. All significances represented as $p < 0.05$, * compared to untreated sample at the same matrix condition, & between oxLDL samples of different cell types at the same matrix condition, and # significant change with collagen concentration. The dotted horizontal line indicates a level of no change.

CD36 is a plasma membrane glycoprotein that binds a diverse array of ligands, including oxLDL [50,51]. As shown in Figure 2B, we found higher CD36 expression solely in M2 macrophage in the absence and presence of oxLDL, whereby a significant up-regulation of CD36 expression could be observed after treatment with oxLDL. The expression of CD36 in THP-1 derived M2 has been reported; these cells were polarized based on a similar protocol [52]. Although M2 showed an increase in both LOX1 and CD36 expression, the amount of oxLDL uptake is lower than the M1 counterpart, which exhibited up-regulation of LOX1. The reason could be on account of M2 being anti-atherosclerotic [13] or because of LDL degradation after CD36-mediated uptake [51]. Although the contribution of LOX1 in the oxLDL uptake is reported to be minimal compared to other receptors [42], an increase of soluble LOX1 can contribute up to 40% in oxLDL uptake [43]. Similar to LOX1, we observed a slight increase in CD36 expression of M2 in the denser matrix after treatment with oxLDL. A report suggested a correlation between vessel stiffening and CD36 expression in endothelial cells [53]. To further understand the contributing role of monocytes and macrophages within the atherosclerotic lesion, we performed a quantitative analysis of their secretome using custom bead-based multiplex ELISA.

3.3. RBP4 Is Up-Regulated by All Cell Types with the Addition of oxLDL and Enhanced by High-Density Matrices for THP-1$_{+LDL}$ and M1$_{+LDL}$

Adipokines retinol-binding protein 4 (RBP4), resistin, and leptin are reported to support the progression of atherosclerosis, while adiponectin has protective actions against plaque formation [54]. These factors are also known to be released along with other pro-inflammatory factors during the development of obesity [55–57], and within adipose tissue, they have been shown to induce inflammation by activating macrophages [58]. While no significant statistical differences were found in adipokines, some distinct qualitative trends were observed, which are discussed below. Clinically, RBP4 is a marker for atherosclerotic-associated cardiovascular disease [59]. In animal models, RBP4 has been found to positively contribute towards atherosclerotic progression and mediate LDL uptake [60]. In our model, we found an increase in RPB4 secretion by all cell types in response to oxLDL (Figure 3A); generally, higher secretions were measured in the denser matrix for THP-1$_{+LDL}$ and M1$_{+LDL}$. It has been demonstrated that RBP4 expression was enhanced in the areas rich in macrophage foam cells in atherosclerotic lesions of aortic specimens from both humans and apolipoprotein E-deficient mice [60], suggesting foam cell-like formation in our biomimetic atherosclerosis models.

Leptin reportedly exacerbates inflammation [61] in low matrix density; our results showed that THP-1$_{+LDL}$ and M0$_{+LDL}$ reduced leptin secretion (Figure 3B) as with resistin (Figure 3C). It is reported that human macrophages secrete resistin on their own, and this contributes to atherosclerosis development directly by causing endothelial and smooth muscle cell (SMC) dysfunction [62,63], potentially increasing the permeability of LDL into adjacent tissue. Only THP-1$_{+LDL}$ showed elevated leptin secretion in denser matrices. Evidence suggests that leptin and resistin may initiate the recruitment of monocytes, macrophages, endothelial cells, and smooth muscle cells towards the atherosclerotic site [64,65]. At site, these cell types all individually progress atherosclerosis, although beyond the scope of this study, co-culture experiments with the above-mentioned cell types with our biomimetic model have to be performed to enhance the understanding of this complex disease. The atheroprotective adiponectin was below the assay's theoretical limit of detection using the bead-based ELISA kit (minimum detectable concentration 41.1 pg/mL) in all cells with and without treatment with oxLDL, potentially due to its short half-life [66]. Overall, with the addition of oxLDL there is an increase of secreted adipokines in the dense matrix, particularly by THP-1$_{+LDL}$ and M1$_{+LDL}$, similarly to what would be expected in an advanced atherosclerotic plaque.

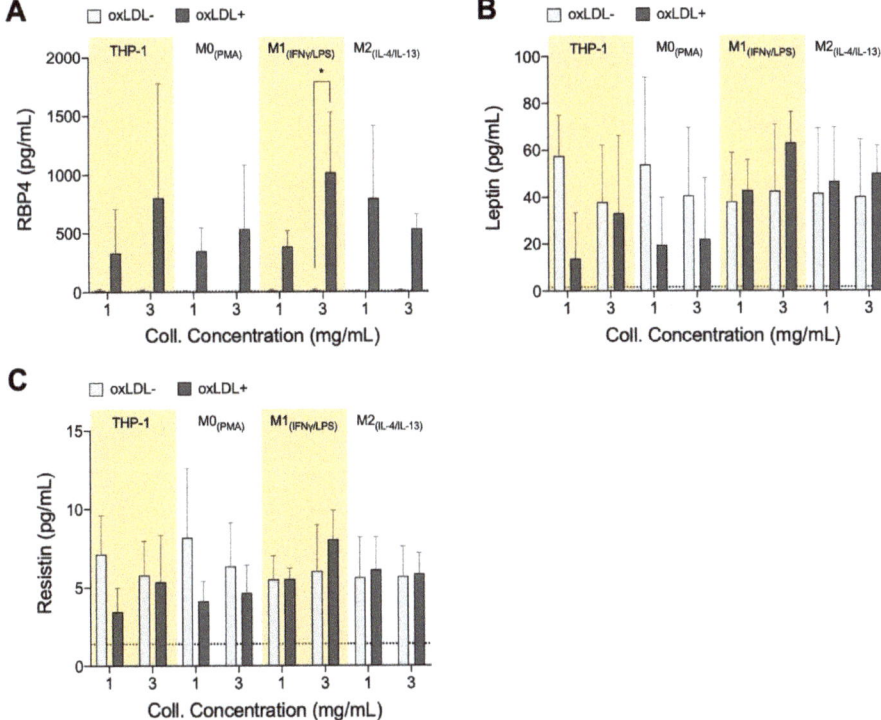

Figure 3. Adipokine secretome from monocytes and macrophages cultured in 3D collagen hydrogels. Box plots of absolute secretion levels of (**A**) RBP4, (**B**) leptin, and (**C**) resistin to observe trends and indicate comparisons that are statistically significant. The dotted line in the box plots marks the lowest detectable concentration of assay. Statistical significance has been determined by two-way ANOVA followed by Tukey's test, and the level of significance is represented as * $p < 0.05$, significantly higher than the untreated sample at the same matrix density condition, no significance otherwise.

3.4. In High-Density Matrices THP-1$_{+LDL}$ and M1$_{+LDL}$ Secretion of Immune Cell Chemoattractants Are Elevated and Suppressed in M2$_{+LDL}$

We measured IP-10, MCP-1, and IL-8 levels from our cell culture system as these are known chemoattractants that are involved in the recruitment of inflammatory cells to the atherosclerotic site [67–69]. Both IP-10 (Figure 4A) and IL-8 (Figure 4B) concentrations are significantly elevated in the dense matrix with M1$_{+LDL}$ compared to the other cell types, whereas the chemoattractants are suppressed with M2$_{+LDL}$. IL-8 recruits cells that participate in acute inflammation [70], while IP-10 is a chemoattractant for immune cells from the adaptive immune system to the atherosclerotic site [71]. It is reviewed in the literature that the adaptive immune system during atherosclerosis changes from a protective to a pathological response, typically when the ratio of effector T-cells to regulatory T-cells increases [72,73]. Therefore, the increased secretion of both IL-8 and IP-10 by M1$_{+LDL}$ in denser collagen matrices, and hence the respective immune cell types, is in response to the stiffer tissue in advanced atherosclerotic plaques.

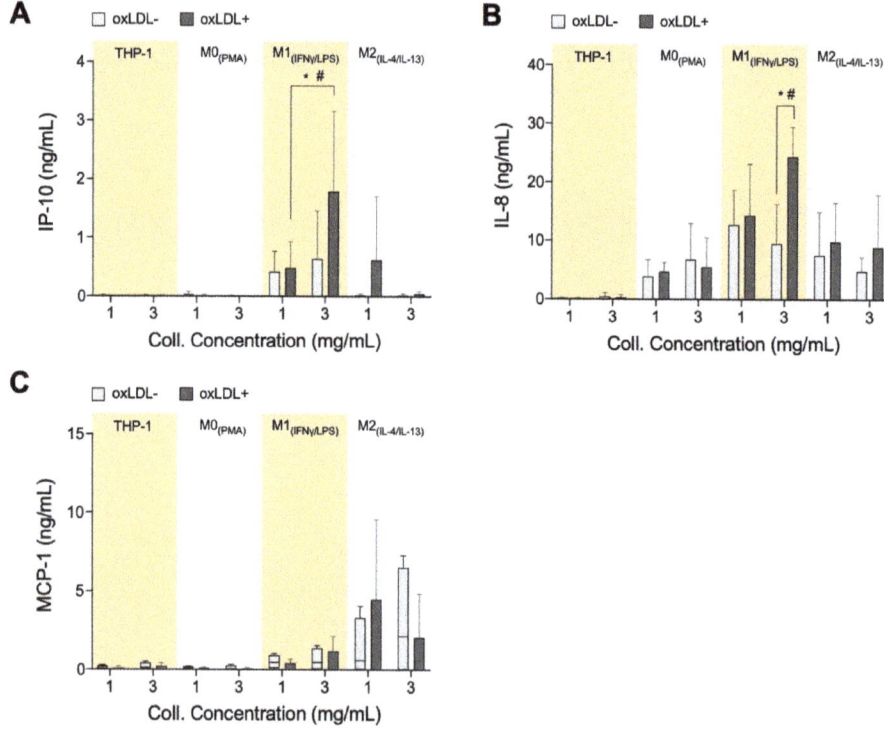

Figure 4. Chemokine secretome from monocytes and macrophages cultured in 3D collagen hydrogels. Box plots of absolute secretion levels of (**A**) IP-10, (**B**) IL-8, and (**C**) MCP-1 to observe trends and indicate comparisons that are statistically significant. The dotted line in box plots marks the lowest detectable concentration of assay. Statistical significance has been determined by two-way ANOVA followed by Tukey's test, and the level of significance is represented as * $p < 0.05$ and # $p < 0.05$ in 3 mg/mL between THP-1$_{+LDL}$, M0$_{+LDL}$, and M2$_{+LDL}$ vs. M1$_{+LDL}$. The dotted horizontal line indicates the lowest detectable limits of the assay.

Unanticipated is the elevated secretion of MCP-1 (Figure 4C) by M2. It is qualitatively highest compared to the other cell types, elevated in low-density matrices and suppressed in denser matrices. Interestingly, both IP-10 and IL-8 in our experiment are secreted at similar concentrations as those measured from atherosclerotic plaques ex vivo [74]. Particularly, IP-10 plays an anti-atherogenic role by inhibiting angiogenesis [75,76]. M2$_{+LDL}$ up-regulation of IP-10, especially in low-density collagen, could signify its potential anti-atherogenic role.

3.5. PDGF-AA, EPO, and M-CSF Are Up-Regulated by Macrophages and VEGF Is Up-Regulated by Monocytes

Endothelial progenitor cells (EPCs) play an important role in the recovery and repair of adult vasculature [77,78]. EPCs reside in bone marrow (BM) and can be signaled to go into circulation to contribute towards the generation of new blood vessels or repair of damaged ones. As atherosclerosis is a result of initial and continual structural and functional endothelial damage, it is expected that EPCs will have an influence on the disease. Clinically, it was observed that high EPC count is a negative predictor of the occurrence of atherosclerotic plaque [79]. Furthermore, recruitment and incorporation of endothelial progenitor cells endogenously into atherosclerotic sites have been shown to attenuate the progression of the disease and mediate vascular repair [80]. For these reasons, we wanted to determine if macrophages within the atherosclerotic microenvironment secrete growth factors to facilitate vascular repair (Figure 5). While differences in growth factor secretion can be observed between cell types, and between treated and untreated cells, no matrix dependence has been observed. There were no significant differences in any of the growth factors, however, the qualitative trends discussed in this section can be discerned from the data.

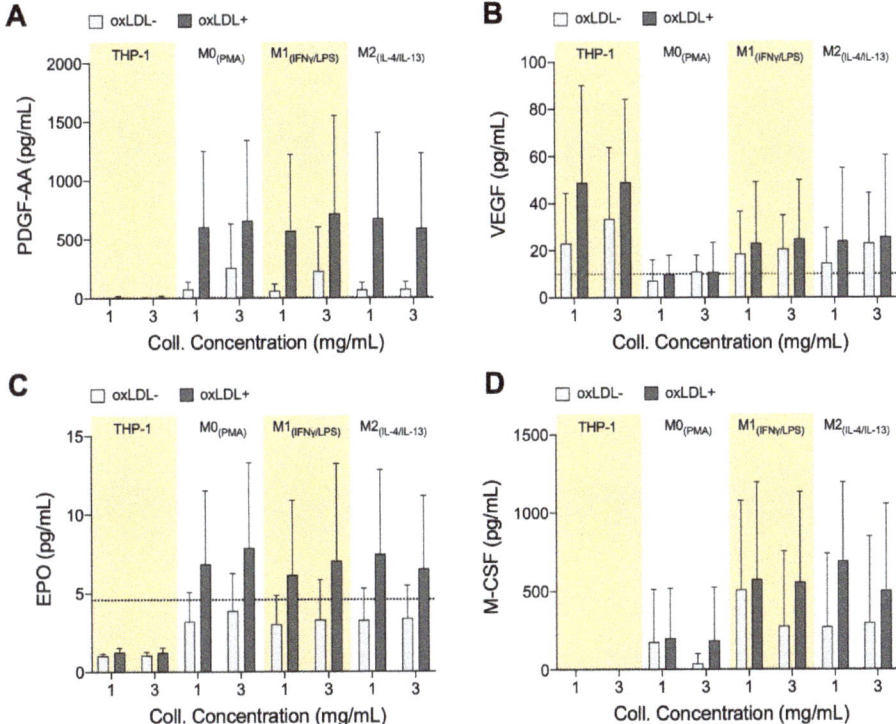

Figure 5. Growth Factor Secretome of monocytes and macrophages cultured in 3D collagen hydrogels. Box plots of absolute secretion levels of (**A**) PDGF-AA, (**B**) VEGF, (**C**) EPO, and (**D**) M-CSF to observe trends. The dotted line in the box plots marks the lowest detectable concentration of assay. Statistical significance has been determined by two-way ANOVA followed by Tukey's test, and the level of significance was set to $p < 0.05$.

Monocytes and all macrophages produce elevated PDGF-AA levels when exposed to oxLDL (Figure 5A). PDGF is known to be involved in the development of new blood vessels [81], and in a recent study, using a mice model, it has been shown that PDGF-AA has the ability to enhance the healing effects of EPCs [82].

The role of VEGF in atherosclerotic plaques is contradictory. Measurement of increased microvessel density in ruptured and unruptured human plaques suggests that VEGF, and other factors that promote blood vessel development, advances atherosclerosis towards destabilization [83]. VEGF is also known to induce the growth of pre-existing vessels as well as to promote the growth of new blood vessels, and therefore this growth factor is also key in vessel repair [84]. From our experiments, oxLDL+ polarized macrophages and monocytes exhibited up-regulation of VEGF secretion (Figure 5B).

EPO stimulates the mobilization of EPCs from bone marrow, animal models, and patients treated with EPO routinely result in increased EPCs in circulation [85,86]. EPO is postulated to also promote homing and differentiation of EPCs at sites of vascular injury [86]. From our results, EPO levels are consistently elevated with the application of oxLDL on macrophages, regardless of their subtype or the matrix density (Figure 5C). EPO, which may inhibit foam cell formation in mice [87], is secreted equally by all our macrophages, whether it has an inhibiting role in our model will need to be further investigated, but initially it could again imply an auto-regulating function of these cells.

M-CSF secretion, like PDGF-AA and EPO, is reserved for macrophages (Figure 5D). Although it has no direct involvement with EPCs, M-CSF has multiple roles in the atherosclerotic microenvironment by regulating migration and recruitment of monocytes and also survival and scavenger activity of macrophages [88]. Although M-CSF is known to induce macrophages into the anti-inflammatory phenotype M2 [89], we observed secretion of this growth factor by $M0_{+LDL}$ and $M1_{+LDL}$, which again could suggest a role in auto-regulating atherosclerosis.

3.6. oxLDL Enhances Expression of CD68 in Monocytes and MHCII Is Enhanced in Dense Matrices for All Cell Types

The consensus is that recruited monocytes will get activated in response to oxLDL into pro-inflammatory macrophages during atherosclerosis [1], we, therefore, analyzed gene expression of *CD68* and *MHCII*. CD68 is a pan-macrophage marker and is up-regulated upon macrophage differentiation [90–92], while MHCII was found to be a marker for pro-inflammatory macrophages [25]. As expected, without oxLDL, as compared to monocytes, we found higher CD68 expression in all macrophages (Figure 6A). In the presence of oxLDL, we found an up-regulation of CD68 in monocytes, which reaffirms the theory of monocyte differentiation into macrophages by oxLDL. No change in CD68 expression could be observed in macrophages with or without oxLDL. This contradicts reports demonstrating the up-regulation of CD68 upon oxLDL treatment in mouse bone-marrow-derived macrophage [93] and also in THP-1-derived M0 macrophages [94]. The discrepancy in CD68 up-regulation upon oxLDL treatment may arise from cell culture dimensionality. Our 3D matrix density did not have any impact on CD68 expression.

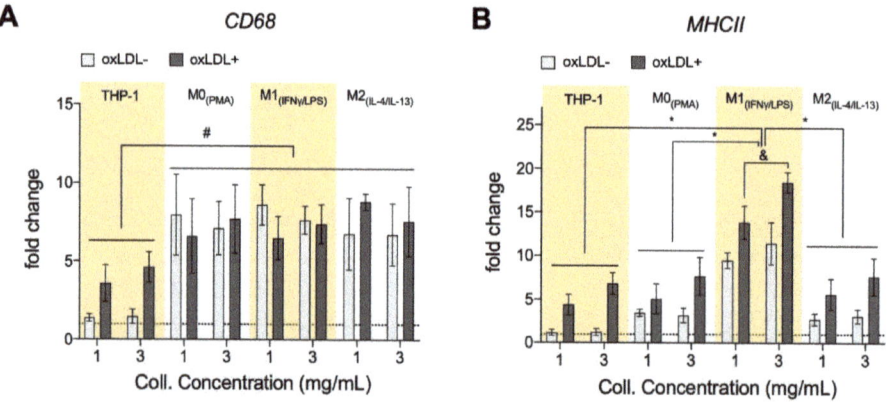

Figure 6. Expression of selected markers of monocytes and macrophages cultured in 3D collagen hydrogels. (**A**) For all cell types, the pan-macrophage marker (CD68) was also increased with the exposure to oxLDL, with THP-1 having the highest fold induction. (**B**) There was an increase in gene expression of the well-acknowledged activation maker (MHCII) in all cell types after exposure to oxLDL. There is also a general increase in expression with increment of collagen hydrogel density (x-axis, 1 (1 mg/mL) → 3 (3 mg/mL)). This correlation of MHCII gene expression with tissue density is statistically significant for THP-1 and M1. All significances represented as $p < 0.05$, * compared to corresponding untreated and treated samples at the same matrix condition, and significant change with collagen concentration and # significant compared to untreated samples at the same matrix conditions. The dotted horizontal line indicates a level of no change.

As we found higher pro-inflammatory adipokine secretion, we hypothesize that oxLDL is capable of influencing a pro-inflammatory macrophage phenotype, which we ascertain through the analysis of the *MHCII* gene expression. As shown in Figure 6B, MHCII is highly expressed in M1 macrophages with higher expression in the dense matrix as corroborated by our previous work [25]. In the presence of oxLDL, monocytes and all macrophages presented enhanced *MHCII* gene expression with the highest in M1. This is supported through the reported oxLDL-mediated uptake activation of spleen tyrosine kinase (SYK) that, in turn, up-regulates MHCII expression in macrophages [95]. Our results suggested that the enhancement of vascular stiffening via matrix density might increase the pro-inflammatory phenotype in response to oxLDL and thus contribute to the progression of atherosclerosis.

4. General Discussion and Conclusions

As mentioned previously, there is a necessity to understand the neglected biochemical contributions by monocytes and macrophages to the atherosclerotic microenvironment. Comprehending the adipokine and growth factor contributions by the various immune cell types within the microenvironment could lead to de novo therapeutic strategies against atherosclerosis. We first revealed that adipokines and growth factors are indeed found in our in vitro model for atherosclerosis. THP-1 monocytes and their derived macrophage subtypes exhibited distinct oxLDL uptake, gene expression, and secretome. As oxLDL and lipid size have no significant differences between cells embedded in low or high matrix densities, we can conclude that several of these differential biological readouts are mediated by the density of the collagen hydrogel-based matrices.

From an adipokine point of view, THP-1$_{+LDL}$ and M0$_{+LDL}$ seem to have a better role in suppressing atherosclerosis in our model, whereby there is down-regulation in adipokines. This is observed predominantly in less dense collagen, which would correspond to earlier stages of atherosclerosis. Moreover, the higher amounts of adipokines in denser matrices reinforces that our denser matrix model produces a cellular reaction similar to more advanced atherogenic stages. In all, with our cell-line-based model of atherosclerosis, adipokines are measurable, and these secretions should be made aware of as they have shown to have an influence on the pro-inflammatory potency of the immune cells in an autocrine manner. In terms of immune cell recruitment, adaptive immune cells are recruited by all macrophage types, with M1$_{+LDL}$ having the greatest influence on their influx into atherosclerotic sites. M2$_{+LDL}$ and M1$_{+LDL}$ actively recruit innate immune cells to atherosclerotic sites, via MCP-1 and IP-10, respectively, also in a matrix density-dependent manner. Finally, the up-regulation of the pro-inflammatory marker MHCII and pan-macrophage marker CD68 by THP-1, confirm that monocytes are differentiating into macrophages in the presence of oxLDL. Furthermore, MHCII shows a trend with collagen concentration, where it is higher in denser collagen matrices. The mechanisms of this matrix-regulation on the cells require further experimentation and are not currently addressed through our study.

The role of M2 is controversial in atherosclerosis, with some studies claiming it could support plaque regression [13], while others argue it supports progression by polarizing towards a pro-inflammatory phenotype instead [35]. Our results suggest that after the removal of activating media and the addition of oxLDL, M2 may adopt a relatively more pro-inflammatory phenotype, in spite of its lower level of oxLDL uptake. This is especially the case in lower density matrices, while in higher density, it seems to retain more of its original phenotype. It is worth noting that after the removal of polarizing media, macrophages are no longer forced into their intended M1 or M2 phenotype. Instead, they are malleable [96], straddling between the M1 and M2 boundaries according to their specific responses to oxLDL and their microenvironment. The same applies to M1 as well as M0, because of their plasticity, their phenotypes are dynamic and non-binary [25], making investigations into atherosclerosis complex, as observed in this study.

From a tissue density perspective, our model represents two different stages of atherosclerotic plaque progression, where a high-density matrix would correspond to a more advanced stage than low density. The main effects of these two different stages of atherosclerosis on each cell type in this study are depicted in Figure 7. Notably, M1$_{+LDL}$ displayed a more pro-inflammatory phenotype in high tissue density, as it is deduced by their secretome and pro-inflammatory marker expression.

While THP-1$_{+LDL}$ suppressed adipokine secretion in low tissue density, the same trend was not found in high tissue density, where RBP4 was greatly increased, which, together with an up-regulation of MHCII, suggests that as atherosclerosis progresses, these cells may adopt a more pro-inflammatory behavior. Moreover, although growth factors were secreted, no matrix dependence was observed. As mentioned above, the role of M2$_{+LDL}$ is somewhat controversial, however, when compared to the other cell types in our model, it appears to adopt a slightly more pro-inflammatory role at the early stages of atherosclerosis supporting plaque progression, and becomes more anti-inflammatory as the atherosclerotic plaque advances, as it is surmised by a decrease of RBP4, IP-10 and MCP-1 in high-density matrices.

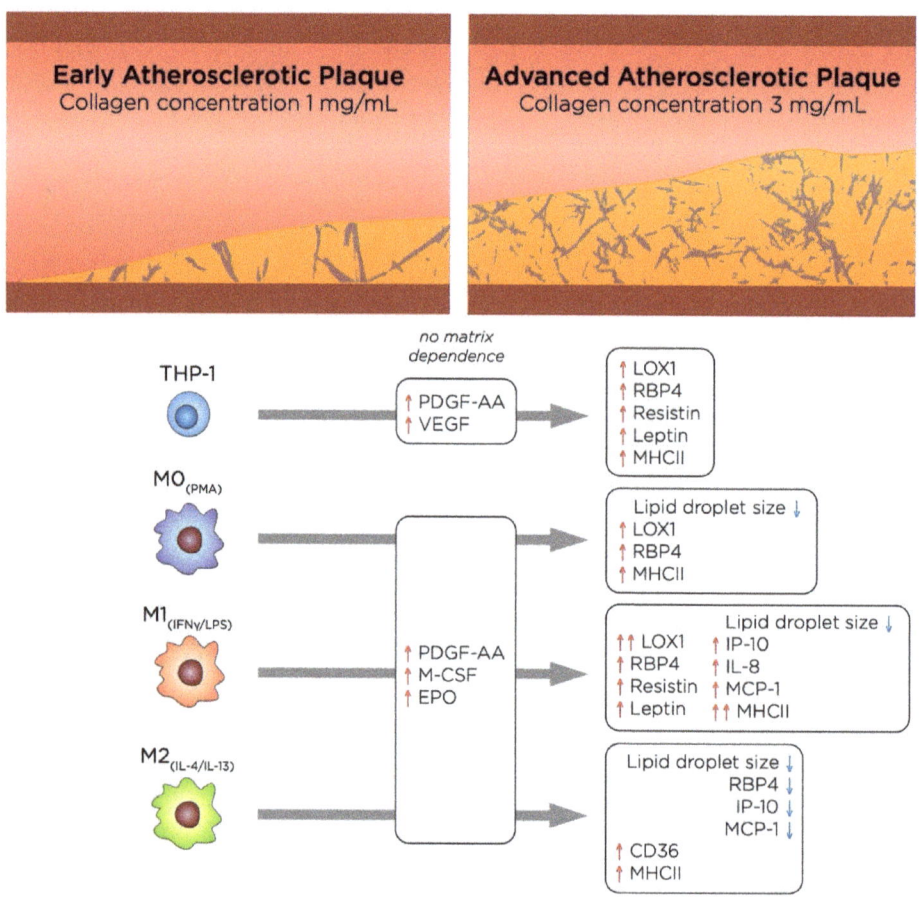

Figure 7. Illustration summarizing the main findings of this study, which highlights the changes undergone by the cells as atherosclerosis progresses.

In conclusion, we have analyzed the oxLDL uptake, secretome, and phenotype of monocytes and macrophages when placed in a physiologically relevant ECM. We have shown that adipokines and growth factors are, in fact, secreted by macrophages and must be taken into considerations for research into atherosclerosis regression and repair. Moreover, our cell-line-based model is able to differentiate monocytes into macrophages after treatment with oxLDL, and these macrophages showed reduced phagocytic capacity and up-regulation of VEGF, which are traits also found in Mox, anti-oxidant macrophages found in murine atherosclerotic plaques, which is induced by oxLDL [97,98]. Future studies to expand this model should include other relevant cells in atherosclerosis, such as SMC and EC, moreover, whether THP-1 derived macrophages have the same phenotype as Mox will also need to be confirmed.

Supplementary Materials: The following are available online at http://www.mdpi.com/2306-5354/7/3/113/s1, Figure S1: Fluorescence assisted cell sorting assessment of LDL uptake by monocytes and macrophages cultured in 3D collagen hydrogels. Table S1: Primer list.

Author Contributions: Conceptualization, A.G.-S., J.S., and J.C.M.T.; methodology, A.G.-S., J.S., W.K.E.M., and L.A.S.; formal analysis, A.G.-S., J.S., and J.C.M.T.; investigation, A.G.-S., W.K.E.M., A.A., L.A.S., J.S., and J.C.M.T.; writing—original draft preparation, A.G.-S., J.S., and J.C.M.T.; writing—review and editing, A.G.-S., W.K.E.M., A.A., L.A.S., J.S., and J.C.M.T.; visualization, A.G.-S., J.S., A.A., and J.C.M.T.; supervision, A.G.-S. and J.C.M.T.; funding acquisition, J.C.M.T. All authors have read and agreed to the published version of the manuscript.

Funding: This research was funded by New York University Abu Dhabi (NYUAD) Faculty Research Fund (AD266) and NYUAD Research Enhancement Fund (RE266 and RE267).

Acknowledgments: The authors would like to acknowledge support by Core Technology Platforms at NYUAD.

Conflicts of Interest: The authors declare no conflict of interest.

References

1. Hansson, G.K.; Hermansson, A. The immune system in atherosclerosis. *Nat. Immunol.* **2011**, *12*, 204–212. [CrossRef]
2. Phipps, R.P. Atherosclerosis: The emerging role of inflammation and the CD40-CD40 ligand system. *Proc. Natl. Acad. Sci. USA* **2000**, *97*, 6930–6932. [CrossRef]
3. Roth, G.A.; Johnson, C.; Abajobir, A.; Abd-Allah, F.; Abera, S.F.; Abyu, G.; Ahmed, M.; Aksut, B.; Alam, T.; Alam, K.; et al. Global, Regional, and National Burden of Cardiovascular Diseases for 10 Causes, 1990 to 2015. *J. Am. Coll. Cardiol.* **2017**, *70*, 1–25. [CrossRef]
4. Gisterå, A.; Hansson, G.K. The immunology of atherosclerosis. *Nat. Rev. Nephrol.* **2017**, *13*, 368–380. [CrossRef]
5. Lusis, A.J. Atherosclerosis. *Nature* **2000**, *407*, 233–241. [CrossRef] [PubMed]
6. Moore, K.J.; Tabas, I. Macrophages in the pathogenesis of atherosclerosis. *Cell* **2011**, *145*, 341–355. [CrossRef] [PubMed]
7. Rader, D.J.; Puré, E. Lipoproteins, macrophage function, and atherosclerosis: Beyond the foam cell? *Cell Metab.* **2005**, *1*, 223–230. [CrossRef]
8. Roma-Lavisse, C.; Tagzirt, M.; Zawadzki, C.; Lorenzi, R.; Vincentelli, A.; Haulon, S.; Juthier, F.; Rauch, A.; Corseaux, D.; Staels, B.; et al. M1 and M2 macrophage proteolytic and angiogenic profile analysis in atherosclerotic patients reveals a distinctive profile in type 2 diabetes. *Diabetes Vasc. Dis. Res.* **2015**, *12*, 279–289. [CrossRef] [PubMed]
9. Barrett, T.J. Macrophages in Atherosclerosis Regression. *Arterioscler. Thromb. Vasc. Biol.* **2020**, *40*, 20–33. [CrossRef]
10. Chistiakov, D.A.; Kashirskikh, D.A.; Khotina, V.A.; Grechko, A.V.; Orekhov, A.N. Immune-Inflammatory Responses in Atherosclerosis: The Role of Myeloid Cells. *J. Clin. Med.* **2019**, *8*, 1798. [CrossRef]
11. De Gaetano, M.; Crean, D.; Barry, M.; Belton, O. M1- and M2-Type Macrophage Responses Are Predictive of Adverse Outcomes in Human Atherosclerosis. *Front. Immunol.* **2016**, *7*, 275. [CrossRef] [PubMed]
12. Pourcet, B.; Staels, B. Alternative macrophages in atherosclerosis: Not always protective! *J. Clin. Investig.* **2018**, *128*, 910–912. [CrossRef]
13. Bi, Y.; Chen, J.; Hu, F.; Liu, J.; Li, M.; Zhao, L. M2 Macrophages as a Potential Target for Antiatherosclerosis Treatment. *Neural Plast.* **2019**, *2019*, 6724903. [CrossRef] [PubMed]
14. Willemsen, L.; de Winther, M.P.J. Macrophage subsets in atherosclerosis as defined by single-cell technologies. *J. Pathol.* **2020**, *250*, 705–714. [CrossRef]
15. Goldberg, I.J.; Sharma, G.; Fisher, E.A. Atherosclerosis: Making a U turn. *Annu. Rev. Med.* **2020**, *71*, 191–201. [CrossRef]

16. Gater, D.L.; Widatalla, N.; Islam, K.; Alraeesi, M.; Teo, J.C.M.; Pearson, Y.E. Quantification of sterol-specific response in human macrophages using automated imaged-based analysis. *Lipids Health Dis.* **2017**, *16*, 242. [CrossRef]
17. Gualtero, D.F.; Lafaurie, G.I.; Fontanilla, M.R. Two-dimensional and three-dimensional models for studying atherosclerosis pathogenesis induced by periodontopathogenic microorganisms. *Mol. Oral Microbiol.* **2018**, *33*, 29–37. [CrossRef] [PubMed]
18. Dorweiler, B.; Torzewski, M.; Dham, M.; Ochsenhirt, V.; Lehr, H.-A.; Lackner, K.J.; Vahl, C.-F. A novel in vitro model for the study of plaque development in atherosclerosis. *Thromb. Haemost.* **2006**, *95*, 182–189. [CrossRef]
19. Robert, J.; Weber, B.; Frese, L.; Emmert, M.Y.; Schmidt, D.; Von Eckardstein, A.; Rohrer, L.; Hoerstrup, S.P. A three-dimensional engineered artery model for in vitro atherosclerosis research. *PLoS ONE* **2013**, *8*, e79821. [CrossRef] [PubMed]
20. Venugopal Menon, N.; Tay, H.M.; Pang, K.T.; Dalan, R.; Wong, S.C.; Wang, X.; Li, K.H.H.; Hou, H.W. A tunable microfluidic 3D stenosis model to study leukocyte-endothelial interactions in atherosclerosis. *APL Bioeng.* **2018**, *2*, 016103. [CrossRef]
21. Mallone, A.; Stenger, C.; Von Eckardstein, A.; Hoerstrup, S.P.; Weber, B. Biofabricating atherosclerotic plaques: In vitro engineering of a three-dimensional human fibroatheroma model. *Biomaterials* **2018**, *150*, 49–59. [CrossRef] [PubMed]
22. Rekhter, M.D. Collagen synthesis in atherosclerosis: Too much and not enough. *Cardiovasc. Res.* **1999**, *41*, 376–384. [CrossRef]
23. Nadkarni, S.K.; Bouma, B.E.; De Boer, J.; Tearney, G.J. Evaluation of collagen in atherosclerotic plaques: The use of two coherent laser-based imaging methods. *Lasers Med. Sci.* **2009**, *24*, 439–445. [CrossRef] [PubMed]
24. Shirwany, N.A.; Zou, M.H. Arterial stiffness: A brief review. *Acta Pharmacol. Sin.* **2010**, *31*, 1267–1276. [CrossRef]
25. Sapudom, J.; Mohamed, W.K.E.; Garcia-Sabaté, A.; Alatoom, A.; Karaman, S.; Mahtani, N.; Teo, J.C. Collagen Fibril Density Modulates Macrophage Activation and Cellular Functions during Tissue Repair. *Bioengineering* **2020**, *7*, 33. [CrossRef] [PubMed]
26. Mundi, S.; Massaro, M.; Scoditti, E.; Carluccio, M.A.; Van Hinsbergh, V.W.M.; Iruela-Arispe, M.L.; De Caterina, R. Endothelial permeability, LDL deposition, and cardiovascular risk factors-A review. *Cardiovasc. Res.* **2018**, *114*, 35–52. [CrossRef] [PubMed]
27. Kim, J.A.; Montagnani, M.; Chandrasekran, S.; Quon, M.J. Role of Lipotoxicity in Endothelial Dysfunction. *Heart Fail. Clin.* **2012**, *8*, 589–607. [CrossRef]
28. Wolf, K.; Alexander, S.; Schacht, V.; Coussens, L.M.; von Andrian, U.H.; van Rheenen, J.; Deryugina, E.; Friedl, P. Collagen-based cell migration models in vitro and in vivo. *Semin. Cell Dev. Biol.* **2009**, *20*, 931–941. [CrossRef]
29. Sapudom, J.; Pompe, T. Biomimetic tumor microenvironments based on collagen matrices. *Biomater. Sci.* **2018**, *6*, 2009–2024. [CrossRef]
30. Sapudom, J.; Rubner, S.; Martin, S.; Kurth, T.; Riedel, S.; Mierke, C.T.; Pompe, T. The phenotype of cancer cell invasion controlled by fibril diameter and pore size of 3D collagen networks. *Biomaterials* **2015**, *52*, 367–375. [CrossRef]
31. Franke, K.; Sapudom, J.; Kalbitzer, L.; Anderegg, U.; Pompe, T. Topologically defined composites of collagen types I and V as in vitro cell culture scaffolds. *Acta Biomater.* **2014**, *10*, 2693–2702. [CrossRef] [PubMed]
32. Sapudom, J.; Alatoom, A.; Mohamed, W.K.E.; Garcia-Sabaté, A.; McBain, I.; Nasser, R.A.; Teo, J.C.M. Dendritic cell immune potency on 2D and in 3D collagen matrices. *Biomater. Sci.* **2020**, *8*, 5106–5120. [CrossRef] [PubMed]
33. Feig, J.E.; Parathath, S.; Rong, J.X.; Mick, S.L.; Vengrenyuk, Y.; Grauer, L.; Young, S.G.; Fisher, E.A. Reversal of hyperlipidemia with a genetic switch favorably affects the content and inflammatory state of macrophages in atherosclerotic plaques. *Circulation* **2011**, *123*, 989–998. [CrossRef] [PubMed]
34. McWhorter, F.Y.; Davis, C.T.; Liu, W.F. Physical and mechanical regulation of macrophage phenotype and function. *Cell. Mol. Life Sci.* **2015**, *72*, 1303–1316. [CrossRef]

35. Van Tits, L.J.H.; Stienstra, R.; van Lent, P.L.; Netea, M.G.; Joosten, L.A.B.; Stalenhoef, A.F.H. Oxidized LDL enhances pro-inflammatory responses of alternatively activated M2 macrophages: A crucial role for Krüppel-like factor 2. *Atherosclerosis* **2011**, *214*, 345–349. [CrossRef]
36. De La Paz Sánchez-Martínez, M.; Blanco-Favela, F.; Mora-Ruiz, M.D.; Chávez-Rueda, A.K.; Bernabe-García, M.; Chávez-Sánchez, L. IL-17-differentiated macrophages secrete pro-inflammatory cytokines in response to oxidized low-density lipoprotein. *Lipids Health Dis.* **2017**, *16*, 196. [CrossRef]
37. Adamson, S.; Leitinger, N. Phenotypic modulation of macrophages in response to plaque lipids. *Curr. Opin. Lipidol.* **2011**, *22*, 335–342. [CrossRef]
38. Chistiakov, D.A.; Bobryshev, Y.V.; Nikiforov, N.G.; Elizova, N.V.; Sobenin, I.A.; Orekhov, A.N. Macrophage phenotypic plasticity in atherosclerosis: The associated features and the peculiarities of the expression of inflammatory genes. *Int. J. Cardiol.* **2015**, *184*, 436–445. [CrossRef]
39. De Paoli, F.; Staels, B.; Chinetti-Gbaguidi, G. Macrophage phenotypes and their modulation in atherosclerosis. *Circ. J.* **2014**, *78*, 1775–1781. [CrossRef]
40. Peled, M.; Nishi, H.; Weinstock, A.; Barrett, T.J.; Zhou, F.; Quezada, A.; Fisher, E.A. A wild-type mouse-based model for the regression of inflammation in atherosclerosis. *PLoS ONE* **2017**, *12*, e173975. [CrossRef]
41. Palanisamy, G.S.; Kirk, N.M.; Ackart, D.F.; Obregón-Henao, A.; Shanley, C.A.; Orme, I.M.; Basaraba, R.J. Uptake and accumulation of oxidized low-density lipoprotein during mycobacterium tuberculosis infection in guinea pigs. *PLoS ONE* **2012**, *7*, e34148. [CrossRef] [PubMed]
42. Kunjathoor, V.V.; Febbraio, M.; Podrez, E.A.; Moore, K.J.; Andersson, L.; Koehn, S.; Rhee, J.S.; Silverstein, R.; Hoff, H.F.; Freeman, M.W. Scavenger Receptors Class A-I/II and CD36 Are the Principal Receptors Responsible for the Uptake of Modified Low Density Lipoprotein Leading to Lipid Loading in Macrophages. *J. Biol. Chem.* **2002**, *277*, 49982–49988. [CrossRef] [PubMed]
43. Kattoor, A.J.; Goel, A.; Mehta, J.L. LOX-1: Regulation, Signaling and Its Role in Atherosclerosis. *Antioxidants* **2019**, *8*, 218. [CrossRef] [PubMed]
44. Aoyama, T.; Sawamura, T.; Furutani, Y.; Matsuoka, R.; Yoshida, M.C.; Fujiwara, H.; Masaki, T. Structure and chromosomal assignment of the human lectin-like oxidized low-density-lipoprotein receptor-1 (LOX-1) gene. *Biochem. J.* **1999**, *339*, 177–184. [CrossRef] [PubMed]
45. N'Guessan, P.D.; Riediger, F.; Vardarova, K.; Scharf, S.; Eitel, J.; Opitz, B.; Slevogt, H.; Weichert, W.; Hocke, A.C.; Schmeck, B.; et al. Statins control oxidized ldl-mediated histone modifications and gene expression in cultured human endothelial cells. *Arterioscler. Thromb. Vasc. Biol.* **2009**, *29*, 380–386. [CrossRef]
46. Xu, S.; Ogura, S.; Chen, J.; Little, P.J.; Moss, J.; Liu, P. LOX-1 in atherosclerosis: Biological functions and pharmacological modifiers. *Cell. Mol. Life Sci.* **2013**, *70*, 2859–2872. [CrossRef]
47. Peled, M.; Fisher, E.A. Dynamic aspects of macrophage polarization during atherosclerosis progression and regression. *Front. Immunol.* **2014**, *5*, 579. [CrossRef]
48. Shioi, A.; Ikari, Y. Plaque calcification during atherosclerosis progression and regression. *J. Atheroscler. Thromb.* **2018**, *25*, 294–303. [CrossRef]
49. Di Gregoli, K.; Somerville, M.; Bianco, R.; Thomas, A.C.; Frankow, A.; Newby, A.C.; George, S.J.; Jackson, C.L.; Johnson, J.L. Galectin-3 Identifies a Subset of Macrophages with a Potential Beneficial Role in Atherosclerosis. *Arterioscler. Thromb. Vasc. Biol.* **2020**, *40*, 1491–1509. [CrossRef]
50. Moore, K.J.; Freeman, M.W. Scavenger receptors in atherosclerosis: Beyond lipid uptake. *Arterioscler. Thromb. Vasc. Biol.* **2006**, *26*, 1702–1711. [CrossRef]
51. Endemann, G.; Stanton, L.W.; Madden, K.S.; Bryant, C.M.; White, R.T.; Protter, A.A. CD36 is a receptor for oxidized low density lipoprotein. *J. Biol. Chem.* **1993**, *268*, 11811–11816. [PubMed]
52. Tang, H.; Husch, J.F.A.; Zhang, Y.; Jansen, J.A.; Yang, F.; van den Beucken, J.J.J.P. Coculture with monocytes/macrophages modulates osteogenic differentiation of adipose-derived mesenchymal stromal cells on poly(lactic-co-glycolic) acid/polycaprolactone scaffolds. *J. Tissue Eng. Regen. Med.* **2019**, *13*, 785–798. [CrossRef] [PubMed]
53. Le Master, E.; Fancher, I.S.; Lee, J.; Levitan, I. Comparative analysis of endothelial cell and sub-endothelial cell elastic moduli in young and aged mice: Role of CD36. *J. Biomech.* **2018**, *76*, 263–268. [CrossRef] [PubMed]
54. Ouchi, N.; Parker, J.L.; Lugus, J.J.; Walsh, K. Adipokines in inflammation and metabolic disease. *Nat. Rev. Immunol.* **2011**, *11*, 85–97. [CrossRef]

55. Xu, X.; Grijalva, A.; Skowronski, A.; Van Eijk, M.; Serlie, M.J.; Ferrante, A.W. Obesity activates a program of lysosomal-dependent lipid metabolism in adipose tissue macrophages independently of classic activation. *Cell Metab.* **2013**, *18*, 816–830. [CrossRef]
56. Boden, G.; Chen, X.; Ruiz, J.; White, J.V.; Rossetti, L. Mechanisms of fatty acid-induced inhibition of glucose uptake. *J. Clin. Investig.* **1994**, *93*, 2438–2446. [CrossRef]
57. Boden, G. Obesity and Free Fatty Acids. *Endocrinol. Metab. Clin. N. Am.* **2008**, *37*, 635–646. [CrossRef]
58. Moraes-Vieira, P.M.; Yore, M.M.; Dwyer, P.M.; Syed, I.; Aryal, P.; Kahn, B.B. RBP4 activates antigen-presenting cells, leading to adipose tissue inflammation and systemic insulin resistance. *Cell Metab.* **2014**, *19*, 512–526. [CrossRef]
59. Silverstein, R.L. Linking Metabolic Dysfunction to Atherosclerosis Via Activation of Macrophage CD36 Gene Transcription by Retinol Binding Protein-4. *Circulation* **2017**, *135*, 1355–1357. [CrossRef]
60. Liu, Y.; Zhong, Y.; Chen, H.; Wang, D.; Wang, M.; Ou, J.S.; Xia, M. Retinol-binding protein-dependent cholesterol uptake regulates macrophage foam cell formation and promotes atherosclerosis. *Circulation* **2017**, *135*, 1339–1354. [CrossRef]
61. Monteiro, L.; Pereira, J.A.d.S.; Palhinha, L.; Moraes-Vieira, P.M.M. Leptin in the regulation of the immunometabolism of adipose tissue-macrophages. *J. Leukoc. Biol.* **2019**, *106*, 703–716. [CrossRef] [PubMed]
62. Jung, H.S.; Park, K.H.; Cho, Y.M.; Chung, S.S.; Cho, H.J.; Cho, S.Y.; Kim, S.J.; Kim, S.Y.; Lee, H.K.; Park, K.S. Resistin is secreted from macrophages in atheromas and promotes atherosclerosis. *Cardiovasc. Res.* **2006**, *69*, 76–85. [CrossRef] [PubMed]
63. Park, H.K.; Kwak, M.K.; Kim, H.J.; Ahima, R.S. Linking resistin, inflammation, and cardiometabolic diseases. *Korean J. Intern. Med.* **2017**, *32*, 239–247. [CrossRef] [PubMed]
64. Curat, C.A.; Miranville, A.; Sengene, C.; Diehl, M.; Tonus, C.; Busse, R.; Bouloumie, A. From Blood Monocytes to Adipose Tissue-Resident Macrophages. *Diabetes* **2004**, *53*, 1285–1292. [CrossRef]
65. Cho, Y.; Lee, S.E.; Lee, H.C.; Hur, J.; Lee, S.; Youn, S.W.; Lee, J.; Lee, H.J.; Lee, T.K.; Park, J.; et al. Adipokine resistin is a key player to modulate monocytes, endothelial cells, and smooth muscle cells, leading to progression of atherosclerosis in rabbit carotid artery. *J. Am. Coll. Cardiol.* **2011**, *57*, 99–109. [CrossRef]
66. Wang, Z.V.; Scherer, P.E. Adiponectin, the past two decades. *J. Mol. Cell Biol.* **2016**, *8*, 93–100. [CrossRef]
67. Lin, J.; Kakkar, V.; Lu, X. Impact of MCP -1 in Atherosclerosis. *Curr. Pharm. Des.* **2014**, *20*, 4580–4588. [CrossRef]
68. Van Den Borne, P.; Quax, P.H.A.; Hoefer, I.E.; Pasterkamp, G. The multifaceted functions of CXCL10 in cardiovascular disease. *Biomed. Res. Int.* **2014**, *2014*, 893106. [CrossRef]
69. Apostolopoulos, J.; Davenport, P.; Tipping, P.G. Interleukin-8 Production by Macrophages from Atheromatous Plaques. *Arterioscler. Thromb. Vasc. Biol.* **1996**, *16*, 1007–1012. [CrossRef]
70. Apostolakis, S.; Vogiatzi, K.; Amanatidou, V.; Spandidos, D.A. Interleukin 8 and cardiovascular disease. *Cardiovasc. Res.* **2009**, *84*, 353–360. [CrossRef]
71. Zernecke, A.; Shagdarsuren, E.; Weber, C. Chemokines in atherosclerosis an update. *Arterioscler. Thromb. Vasc. Biol.* **2008**, *28*, 1897–1908. [CrossRef]
72. Wolf, D.; Ley, K. Immunity and Inflammation in Atherosclerosis. *Circ. Res.* **2019**, *124*, 315–327. [CrossRef]
73. Tabas, I.; Lichtman, A.H. Monocyte-Macrophages and T Cells in Atherosclerosis. *Immunity* **2017**, *47*, 621–634. [CrossRef] [PubMed]
74. Lebedeva, A.; Vorobyeva, D.; Vagida, M.; Ivanova, O.; Felker, E.; Fitzgerald, W.; Danilova, N.; Gontarenko, V.; Shpektor, A.; Vasilieva, E.; et al. Ex vivo culture of human atherosclerotic plaques: A model to study immune cells in atherogenesis. *Atherosclerosis* **2017**, *267*, 90–98. [CrossRef] [PubMed]
75. Camaré, C.; Pucelle, M.; Nègre-Salvayre, A.; Salvayre, R. Angiogenesis in the atherosclerotic plaque. *Redox Biol.* **2017**, *12*, 18–34. [CrossRef] [PubMed]
76. Strieter, R.M.; Burdick, M.D.; Gomperts, B.N.; Belperio, J.A.; Keane, M.P. CXC chemokines in angiogenesis. *Cytokine Growth Factor Rev.* **2005**, *16*, 593–609. [CrossRef]
77. Du, F.; Zhou, J.; Gong, R.; Huang, X.; Pansuria, M.; Virtue, A.; Li, X.; Wang, H.; Yang, X.-F. Endothelial progenitor cells in atherosclerosis. *Front. Biosci.* **2012**, *17*, 2327–2349. [CrossRef]

78. Yang, J.X.; Pan, Y.Y.; Wang, X.X.; Qiu, Y.G.; Mao, W. Endothelial progenitor cells in age-related vascular remodeling. *Cell Transplant.* **2018**, *27*, 786–795. [CrossRef]
79. Fadini, G.P.; Sartore, S.; Albiero, M.; Baesso, I.; Murphy, E.; Menegolo, M.; Grego, F.; De Kreutzenberg, S.V.; Tiengo, A.; Agostini, C.; et al. Number and function of endothelial progenitor cells as a marker of severity for diabetic vasculopathy. *Arterioscler. Thromb. Vasc. Biol.* **2006**, *26*, 2140–2146. [CrossRef]
80. Dimmeler, S.; Zeiher, A.M. Vascular repair by circulating endothelial progenitor cells: The missing link in atherosclerosis? *J. Mol. Med.* **2004**, *82*, 671–677. [CrossRef]
81. Raica, M.; Cimpean, A.M. Platelet-derived growth factor (PDGF)/PDGF receptors (PDGFR) axis as target for antitumor and antiangiogenic therapy. *Pharmaceuticals* **2010**, *3*, 572–599. [CrossRef] [PubMed]
82. Wu, L.W.; Chen, W.L.; Huang, S.M.; Chan, J.Y.H. Platelet-derived growth factor-AA is a substantial factor in the ability of adipose-derived stem cells and endothelial progenitor cells to enhance wound healing. *FASEB J.* **2019**, *33*, 2388–2395. [CrossRef] [PubMed]
83. Van Der Veken, B.; De Meyer, G.; Martinet, W. Inhibition of VEGF receptor signaling attenuates intraplaque angiogenesis and plaque destabilization in a mouse model of advanced atherosclerosis. *Atherosclerosis* **2017**, *263*, e33–e34. [CrossRef]
84. Korn, C.; Augustin, H.G. Mechanisms of Vessel Pruning and Regression. *Dev. Cell* **2015**, *34*, 5–17. [CrossRef] [PubMed]
85. Yip, H.K.; Tsai, T.H.; Lin, H.S.; Chen, S.F.; Sun, C.K.; Leu, S.; Yuen, C.M.; Tan, T.Y.; Lan, M.Y.; Liou, C.W.; et al. Effect of erythropoietin on level of circulating endothelial progenitor cells and outcome in patients after acute ischemic stroke. *Crit. Care* **2011**, *15*, R40. [CrossRef] [PubMed]
86. Xu, Y.; Tian, Y.; Wei, H.J.; Chen, J.; Dong, J.F.; Zacharek, A.; Zhang, J.N. Erythropoietin increases circulating endothelial progenitor cells and reduces the formation and progression of cerebral aneurysm in rats. *Neuroscience* **2011**, *181*, 292–299. [CrossRef]
87. Lu, K.Y.; Ching, L.C.; Su, K.H.; Yu, Y.B.; Kou, Y.R.; Hsiao, S.H.; Huang, Y.C.; Chen, C.Y.; Cheng, L.C.; Pan, C.C.; et al. Erythropoietin suppresses the formation of macrophage foam cells: Role of liver X receptor α. *Circulation* **2010**, *121*, 1828–1837. [CrossRef]
88. Viktorinova, A. Potential Clinical Utility of Macrophage Colony-stimulating Factor, Monocyte Chemotactic Protein-1, and Myeloperoxidase in Predicting Atherosclerotic Plaque Instability. *Discov. Med.* **2019**, *28*, 237–245.
89. Zhang, Y.H.; He, M.; Wang, Y.; Liao, A.H. Modulators of the balance between M1 and M2 macrophages during pregnancy. *Front. Immunol.* **2017**, *8*, 120. [CrossRef]
90. Yang, J.; Zhang, L.; Yu, C.; Yang, X.F.; Wang, H. Monocyte and macrophage differentiation: Circulation inflammatory monocyte as biomarker for inflammatory diseases. *Biomark. Res.* **2014**, *2*, 1. [CrossRef]
91. Gordon, S.; Mantovani, A. Diversity and plasticity of mononuclear phagocytes. *Eur. J. Immunol.* **2011**, *41*, 2470–2472. [CrossRef] [PubMed]
92. Williams, K.C.; Kim, W.-K. Editorial: Identification of in vivo markers for human polarized macrophages: A need that's finally met. *J. Leukoc. Biol.* **2015**, *98*, 449–450. [CrossRef] [PubMed]
93. Bisgaard, L.S.; Mogensen, C.K.; Rosendahl, A.; Cucak, H.; Nielsen, L.B.; Rasmussen, S.E.; Pedersen, T.X. Bone marrow-derived and peritoneal macrophages have different inflammatory response to oxLDL and M1/M2 marker expression—Implications for atherosclerosis research. *Sci. Rep.* **2016**, *6*, 35234. [CrossRef] [PubMed]
94. Ramprasad, M.P.; Terpstra, V.; Kondratenko, N.; Quehenberger, O.; Steinberg, D. Cell surface expression of mouse macrosialin and human CD68 and their role as macrophage receptors for oxidized low density lipoprotein. *Proc. Natl. Acad. Sci. USA* **1996**, *93*, 14833–14838. [CrossRef] [PubMed]
95. Choi, S.H.; Gonen, A.; Diehl, C.J.; Kim, J.; Almazan, F.; Witztum, J.L.; Miller, Y.I. SYK regulates macrophage MHC-II expression via activation of autophagy in response to oxidized LDL. *Autophagy* **2015**, *11*, 785–795. [CrossRef] [PubMed]
96. Witzel, I.-I.; Nasser, R.; Garcia-Sabaté, A.; Sapudom, J.; Ma, C.; Chen, W.; Teo, J.C.M. Deconstructing Immune Microenvironments of Lymphoid Tissues for Reverse Engineering. *Adv. Healthc. Mater.* **2018**, *8*, 1801126. [CrossRef]

97. Kadl, A.; Meher, A.K.; Sharma, P.R.; Lee, M.Y.; Doran, A.C.; Johnstone, S.R.; Elliott, M.R.; Gruber, F.; Han, J.; Chen, W.; et al. Identification of a novel macrophage phenotype that develops in response to atherogenic phospholipids via Nrf2. *Circ. Res.* **2010**, *107*, 737–746. [CrossRef]
98. Vinchi, F.; Muckenthaler, M.U.; Da Silva, M.C.; Balla, G.; Balla, J.; Jeney, V. Atherogenesis and iron: From epidemiology to cellular level. *Front. Pharmacol.* **2014**, *5*, 94. [CrossRef]

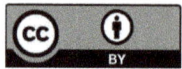

© 2020 by the authors. Licensee MDPI, Basel, Switzerland. This article is an open access article distributed under the terms and conditions of the Creative Commons Attribution (CC BY) license (http://creativecommons.org/licenses/by/4.0/).

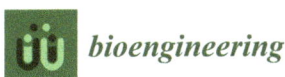

Review

Recent Advancements in 3D Printing and Bioprinting Methods for Cardiovascular Tissue Engineering

Foteini K. Kozaniti *,†, Despoina Nektaria Metsiou †, Aikaterini E. Manara, George Athanassiou and Despina D. Deligianni

Laboratory of Biomechanics & Biomedical Engineering, Department of Mechanical Engineering & Aeronautics, University of Patras, 26504 Patras, Greece; metsiou.betty@gmail.com (D.N.M.); kmanara@upatras.gr (A.E.M.); gathan@mech.upatras.gr (G.A.); deliyian@upatras.gr (D.D.D.)
* Correspondence: fkozaniti@upatras.gr
† The first two authors contributed equally to the project.

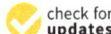

Citation: Kozaniti, F.K.; Metsiou, D.N.; Manara, A.E.; Athanassiou, G.; Deligianni, D.D. Recent Advancements in 3D Printing and Bioprinting Methods for Cardiovascular Tissue Engineering. *Bioengineering* **2021**, *8*, 133. https://doi.org/10.3390/bioengineering8100133

Academic Editors: Efstathios Michalopoulos and Panagiotis Mallis

Received: 21 August 2021
Accepted: 24 September 2021
Published: 27 September 2021

Publisher's Note: MDPI stays neutral with regard to jurisdictional claims in published maps and institutional affiliations.

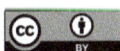

Copyright: © 2021 by the authors. Licensee MDPI, Basel, Switzerland. This article is an open access article distributed under the terms and conditions of the Creative Commons Attribution (CC BY) license (https://creativecommons.org/licenses/by/4.0/).

Abstract: Recent decades have seen a plethora of regenerating new tissues in order to treat a multitude of cardiovascular diseases. Autografts, xenografts and bioengineered extracellular matrices have been employed in this endeavor. However, current limitations of xenografts and exogenous scaffolds to acquire sustainable cell viability, anti-inflammatory and non-cytotoxic effects with anti-thrombogenic properties underline the requirement for alternative bioengineered scaffolds. Herein, we sought to encompass the methods of biofabricated scaffolds via 3D printing and bioprinting, the biomaterials and bioinks recruited to create biomimicked tissues of cardiac valves and vascular networks. Experimental and computational designing approaches have also been included. Moreover, the in vivo applications of the latest studies on the treatment of cardiovascular diseases have been compiled and rigorously discussed.

Keywords: cardiovascular disease; tissue engineering; 3D bioprinting; cell therapy

1. Introduction

Cardiovascular disease (CVD) is the leading cause of morbidity and mortality globally; according to World Health Organization (WHO) more than 17.9 million people die from such causes every year—an estimated 31% of all deaths worldwide [1]. Simultaneously, the estimated healthcare cost for cardiovascular disease in Europe reaches to 169 billion € [2]. It is well established that more than 80% of CVD deaths occur in low-and middle-income countries compared to high-income countries [3,4]. Therefore, the need to reduce the economic burden is not debatable. CVD includes a wide group of complex disorders, namely peripheral arterial disease (PAD), coronary heart disease (CHD), cerebrovascular disease and rheumatic heart disease [2].

Current high-cost therapies include conventional tissue engineering, cell therapy and medical approaches [5,6]. In valve repairment, autografts are widely used by harvesting from autologous cell sources, namely parts of a patient's body with the advent of low risk of thromboembolism and prosthetic valve infection [7]. The end stage heart failure is treated by allografting a heart from a donor, while some valve replacement surgeries employ bovine or porcine heart valves. Xenografts, though, impute other undesirable properties, including cytotoxicity and calcification [8]. Conclusively, the aforementioned grafts have their set of drawbacks, including shortage of donor organs, mechanical mismatches, anticoagulation therapy and immune rejection [9]. Synthetic valves and vascular grafts can also be implanted to treat CVD; however, the high structural durability and low rate of re-operation is outweighed by the increased risk of anticoagulation complications in patients with long life expectancy [10]. Small-diameter vascular grafts (SDVGs) constructed from synthetic polymers and decellularized matrices are promising in the field of reconstructive surgery; however, further evaluation and in vivo implementations are mandatory in order to be applied to therapeutic approaches in CVD [2].

Therefore, one showcasing solution will be the overarching focus on identifying alternative tissue treatments that preserve natural tissue without deleterious side effects.

The increased demand on recovery of damaged cardiovascular tissues in combination with the demand for low-cost but effective constructions, heralds new methods in tissue engineering [11]. Three-dimensional (3D) printing and bioprinting are the recent promising methods that successfully regenerate various organs, scaffolds and blood vessels, which can be used for replacing partly or thoroughly natural organs in the human body [12,13]. With the advent of additive manufacturing, 3D bioprinting technology employs a layer-by-layer approach which enables precise control over multiple compositions (biomaterials) and spatial distributions (cells) resulting in architectural construction accuracy [14]. Biomaterials that have been employed in 3D printing for cardiovascular tissue engineering are major natural or synthetic hydrogels, or decellularized matrices in order to mimic the dense vascular network that supports the cardiac tissue, by providing an interconnected porous network that enables cells to migrate, proliferate and receive vital nutrients and adequate oxygen supply [2,11,15,16]. This takes into consideration the survival distance limitation for cells which is no further than $100 \div 200$ μm away from blood vessels [17]. Alginate and collagen are the most commonly used hydrogels in bioprinting following gelatin methacrylate, fibrinogen and gelatin [18]. Cell viability, proliferation and morphology after printing are crucially affected by characteristics of the selected bioink [19]. The challenge of bioink design is the improvement of printability without detracting cell viability [20]. Biomaterial-based hydrogels are capable of cell encapsulation. The major cell types that integrate the cardiac tissue are cardiomyocytes, endothelial cells, smooth muscle cells and fibroblasts. Furthermore, computational simulation with a patient's anatomical data and features is compulsory for an integrated patient-specific bioprinted construct.

The current review article, briefly outlines the basic principles and growing applications of 3D bioprinting, highlighting key developments and in vivo implementation in the field of cardiovascular tissue engineering. More specifically, 3D-printing definitions are presented, and the 3D construct stages of manufacturing are investigated followed by the computational and experimental designing approach. In addition, different techniques of bioprinting and constitution of the inks are presented thoroughly. In closing, this review outlines recent innovative in vivo studies on 3D bioprinted applicable therapeutic approaches in CVD.

2. From 3D Printing to the New Era of 3D Bioprinting

2.1. Three-Dimensional Printing—Additive Manufacturing

The terms "3D printing" and "additive manufacturing" are usually confused. According to the American Society for Testing and Materials (ASTM), additive manufacturing is the process of joining materials using 3D model data layer by layer in contrast to subtractive manufacturing methodologies, such as traditional machining [21,22], whereas "3D printing" is defined as object fabrication through the deposition of a material with the help of a print head, nozzle or another printer technology [21]. The two terms are often used synonymously, especially considering they are low end in price and/or overall capability [21].

Moroni et al. tried to define "3D printing" based on the appearance of the printing process with cell-laden inks [23]. According to them, in this additive manufacturing technology a jet of binder is directed at a powder bed to define a pattern. A slice of solid material is formed after the binding of the solvent to the powder. A new layer of powder is set and by repeating this process the scaffold is build layer by layer. This definition was based on the first patent for 3D printing of Sachs et al., in which a binder solution was deposited in a powder bed according to a Computer Aided Design (CAD) model [24]. However, in the recent research of Marti et al., 3D printing is referred as the process of additive production of 3D objects, which starts from a 3D digital model [25]. Thus, the term 3D printing is still used instead of additive manufacturing for the sake of simplicity.

Computational Stage—Preparation of 3D Printing

Computational methods are widely used to study tissue engineered constructs. However, the entrance of computer designing is essential in the field of tissue bioengineering due to personalized medicine. The main idea is to produce a specialized human part for each specific patient, thus contributing to a more efficient and low-cost tissue engineering [26]. The main purpose of this strategy is to create a tissue engineered scaffold with similar mechanical and biological properties concerning the defective tissue [20]. This procedure includes the following steps.

The tissue defect is digitally visualized using imaging machines, particularly CT scan (Computer Tomography scan), MRI (Magnetic Resonance Imaging) and ultrasound scan. The next step is to create a scaffold that readily supports the formation of the new tissue. The architecture of the scaffold can be meticulously designed using Computer Aided Design (CAD), a feasible way to manipulate the design parameters of tissue porosity, dimensions and biological-related properties. The scaffold can now be integrated into the 3D model of the defective tissue. Subsequently, bioink will be fabricated by assessing the proper materials, the cell types and bioactive molecules, and the location and requirements of the injured area of the patient. Eventually, using bioprinting technology the cell seeded construct can be manufactured and then placed in a cell culture or implanted directly into the patient [27].

Three-dimensional printing enables the precise fabrication of computationally designed scaffolds with increased accuracy, flexibility and reproducibility. These methods allow scientists to conduct low-cost parametric studies in order to create the most functional construct for the addressed medical issue. The structural design and the mechanical behavior under different conditions of the small diameter composite vascular grafts can easily be optimized by using computational methods.

Computational methods integrate the 3D printing methods and provide the following advantages:

- more accurate techniques to model the scaffolds (e.g., image-based modelling using micro-CT), as an extra feature to reinforce the personalised medicine
- more detailed mechanobiological models to simulate different types of tissues
- more similar to in vivo conditions simulations of the scaffold's properties and behavior under different conditions
- minimized size effect during scaffold modelling
- reduced experimental expenses (elimination of trial-and-error techniques to find the suitable scaffold)
- simultaneous estimation of the scaffold degradation and tissue regeneration in the time-dependent simulations [28,29].

A crucial issue in 3D printed tissue engineering is that the new formatted tissue may not develop adequate vascularisation for long-term survival [12]. The 3D printed construct must provide nutrients and growth factors to cells in order to proliferate [15]. However, key parameters that affect the vascularisation and need to be overcome are the shear stress from blood flow and the wall shear stress [13]. A feasible way to anticipate this challenge is through computational fluid dynamics simulations. Nowadays, personalized medicine is widely applicable and therefore three-dimensional hemodynamic simulations could contribute to the diagnosis of CVDs in order to demonstrate the needs of each patient [30]. Conclusively, flow simulations support the design and additive manufacturing techniques to produce patient-specific 3D printed biodegradable scaffolds, thus being tailored to the individual patient based on their predicted post-surgical response [31].

2.2. Bioprinting

Three-dimensional bioprinting has emerged as an advanced and novel process in the field of tissue engineering and regenerative medicine. Notably, researchers' interest in bioprinting is also evident in their efforts to define the term. According to Groll et al., Moroni et al. and Lee et al., bioprinting could be defined as the production of bio-engineered structures through computer-aided transfer processes in order to pattern and assemble living and non-living materials with a prescribed 2D or 3D organization [32–34].

Currently, the use of biomaterials in regenerative medicine and cardiovascular engineering faces challenges, including host inflammatory responses, immunogenicity, biomaterial degradation and toxicity of degradation products, that may affect the long-term function of the engineered tissue construct [35–37]. Therefore, the innovative biomaterial-free method of bioprinting is gaining attention in the scientific society.

Three-dimensional bioprinting has been expected to be a promising method in tissue engineering because of the ability to control precisely the geometry and the amount of biomaterials during construct fabrication [37]. More specifically, this technique can fully incorporate cells into hydrogels that satisfactorily mimic the microenvironment of the extracellular matrix (ECM) and directly print onto the targeted host location [38]. In cardiovascular engineering there are multilateral problems that need to be overcome in order to achieve an integrated 3D bioprinted model [39,40].

Cell viability and vascularization of printed tissues are key factors which determine the effectiveness of bioprinted tissues. Another impediment that needs to be overcome is the promotion of mass transfer of nutrients and oxygen into bioprinted scaffolds, including adhesion molecules and factors that induce angiogenesis [41]. The vascular tissues need substitutes with specific physical characteristics. For example, high stiffness is not favourable like in the cases of bone and cartilage tissues. On the contrary, vascular substitutes must be malleable enough to be shaped correctly in order to regenerate vessels [18]. A schematic representation of the bioprinting process and most recruited bioprinters is illustrated in Figure 1.

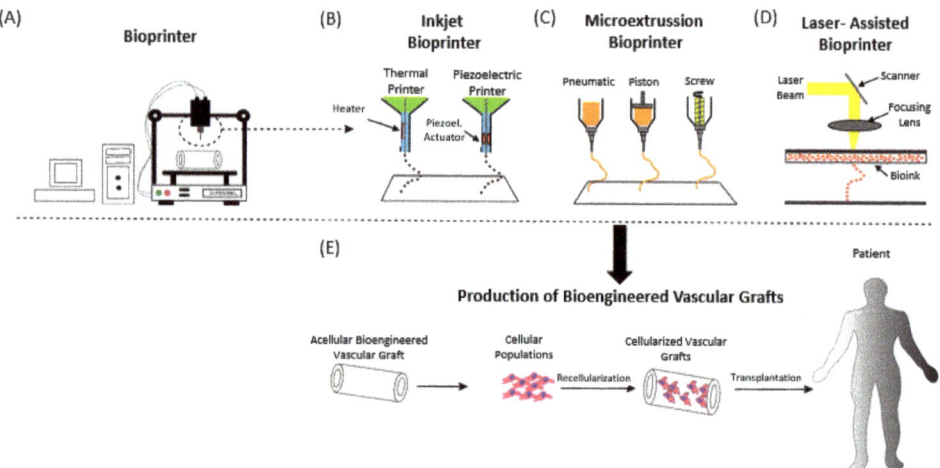

Figure 1. Schematic representation of bioprinters. (**A**) Development of bioengineered vascular grafts with computer assisted software. Different types of bioprinters (**B**), microextrusion bioprinter (**C**) and laser-assisted bioprinter (**D**). (**E**) Production and transplantation of bioengineered vascular grafts. Piezoel: Piezoelectric.

2.2.1. Bioprinting Methods

Several studies and reviews conclude that there are three main types of bioprinting modalities: Droplet-based, extrusion-based and laser-based techniques. [14,42]. Herein, the widely applicable techniques with their set of benefits and drawbacks are briefly introduced in Table 1.

Droplet-Inkjet

The droplet or inkjet-based printing takes place when a bioink solution is forced under pressure and ejected as droplets through a nozzle onto an electronically controlled stage as a result of thermal or acoustic forces [14,43,44]. This heuristic technology favors the precise control of injected cells, growth factors, genes and drugs

The high resolution of the droplet-inkjet construct enables the control of the geometry and scaffold size, whilst the accuracy of cell positioning is an important advantage of the injection method. Moreover, this method is widely used in the case of blood vessels, due to the high-speed printing and the cost-effectiveness construction [14].

Drawbacks of this method include bioink materials with microcarriers, fragments and highly viscous hydrogels that can accumulate within the nozzle and block the flow [45]. Overall, controlling the number of cells to be encapsulated in a single droplet remains the basic challenge of this method [27].

In the Christensen et al. study, vascular-like cellular structures with horizontal and vertical bifurcations were successfully introduced using a liquid support-based inkjet, while the high post-printing fibroblast's cell viability of printed cellular tubes was also reported [46]. Another study introduced a 3D "half-heart" scaffold with connected ventricles printed via an inkjet-based method, where mammalian cardiac cells remained viable with adequate elastic moduli and tensile strength [47].

Extrusion

In extrusion-based bioprinting, a melted polymeric filament or a cell supportive gel can be deposited. The term fused deposition modeling (FDM) is usually used to describe the first way in which a group of polymers of polycaprolactone (PCL), polyurethane (PU) and polylactic acid (PLA) can be extruded. Another way of extruding is the deposition of cell-free or cell-laden hydrogels [14]. For successful construction of vascular networks, researchers introduced and designed coaxial nozzles [48].

Extrusion-based bioprinting is regarded as the most practicable method since the vertical configuration is considered. Nevertheless, the induced shear stress during the printing procedure, often leads to cell death [27]. Moreover, increased shear stress can also lead to a loss of structural integrity regarding the used material, and therefore, the necessity of hydrogels which can regain the mechanical integrity is imperative [49].

According to Tabriz et al., the extrusion technique enables the possibility of bioprinting live human cells with an increased post bioprinting cell survival rate. In their study, alginate hydrogels were formulated with tunable mechanical properties to create straight tubular 3D hydrogel structures with diameters from 7.5 to 20 mm [50].

Furthermore, bioprinting of small diameter vascular grafts through coaxial extrusion possess the advantage of the simultaneous deposition of manifold materials in concentric needles [51]. Intricate multilayered 3D perfusable hollow tubes, with reported diameters 0.5 to 1.5 mm have been manufactured via coaxial nozzle [48]. In the Zhang et al. research, a coaxial nozzle system was used to print vasculature conduits with an outer diameter of 1 mm approximately, and with increased mechanical properties and bioprintability [52]. In their work, human umbilical vein smooth muscle cells (HUVSMCs), were encapsulated in sodium alginate, showed an initial low cell proliferation rate, following though an increased cell viability in prolonged in vitro cell culture.

Laser

In the stereolithography apparatus (SLA), a source of high-power laser solidifies a liquid resin. In a bath full of resin, the light source can produce the desired pattern [20,53]. Superior printability and cell encapsulation capacity have been reported in the biodegradable hydrogel construct in the study of Elomaa et al. [54]. Gaebel et al. [55] introduced cardiac patches for the treatment of myocardial infarction, where cardiac patch was seeded with human umbilical vein endothelial cells and human MSC, improved wound healing and functional preservation.

The main advantage of this method is the fidelity of the achieved geometries. Complex patterns can be manufactured with high resolution, like vascular networks with wide range scales (50–250 µm) [14,56]. The contactless procedure of laser-based bioprinting prevent cells from facing mechanical stresses; thus, high cell viability is expected [53].

The disadvantage of the method is the necessity of photosensitive materials, and hence the selection of bioniks is limited [14,23]. Furthermore, the prerequisite of incorporating a cell type into a hydrogel restricts other possible bioinks [23]. In addition, the cost of the laser diodes is usually higher than its counterparts (nozzles). Moreover, future research could reveal the side effects in cells after the laser exposure during the manufacturing procedure [53].

Table 1. Advantages and limitations of 3D bioprinting techniques for CVD treatment.

	Droplet-Inkjet	Extrusion	Laser	References
Advantages	Increased resolution and speed printing, accuracy of cell positioning, cost-effectiveness construction	Highly viscous bioinks, increased cell density, free-shape structures, most practicable method (as for the vertical configuration)	Fidelity of the achieved geometries, raised cell viability, high resolution complex patterns	[14,27,43,44,57] [48,49] [23,53,56]
Drawbacks	Low viscosity bioinks, induced mechanical forces to cells, inadequate structural integrity and cell encapsulation, use of toxic crosslinkers	Decreased resolution, cell death and degreased structural integrity due to induced shear stress	Limitation of bionics, high cost due to laser diodes, longtime of printing	[14,27,43,44,57] [48,49] [23,53,56]
Bioinks	Alginate	Alginate	Alginate, hyaluronic acid-based solutions, poly-ethylene glycol diacrylate (PEGDA) and poly-(ε-caprolactone) (PCL)	[46,47] [27,50] [54,56,58,59]
Cell type	NIH3 T3 mouse fibroblasts, mammalian cardiac cells	Human glioma U87-MG	human umbilical vein endothelial cells (HUVEC) and human MSC (hMSC)	[46,47] [27,50] [54–56,58,59]
CVD application	Branched tubes with 3 mm diameter [46], Cardiac phaedo tissues ("half heart")	Straight tubes with 7.5–20 mm diameter	Cardiac patch, tissue engineering constructs [55,56,58], branched tubes with 3 mm inner diameter	[47] [27,50] [54,59]

2.2.2. Biomaterials and Inks

Biomaterials

The materials that can be used in the 3D printing technique can be organic or inorganic. The inorganic inks could be categorized into metals, ceramics and glass-ceramics, and the organic ones into thermoplastic and hydrogels [20]. Titanium, cobalt-chrome, stainless steel and magnesium are some of the metallic biomaterials used. Calcium phosphates like hydroxyapatite, brushite and monetite belong in ceramics. In the glass-ceramics category, bioglass, such as silicon dioxide, calcium oxide, sodium oxide and phosphorous pentoxide, is included. As for the organic category, poly-lactic acid (PLA), polyglycolic acid (PGA) and polycaprolactone (PCL) are some of the most frequently used thermoplastics. The category of hydrogels can be divided into synthetic (poly ethylene glycol—PEG; poly vinyl alcohol—PVA; or poly acrylic acid—PAA), semi-synthetic (like derivates of hyaluronic acid, elastin and collagen) and natural (e.g., polynucleotides, polysaccharides and polypeptides) [20].

Bioinks

According to Moroni et al., material (s) and biological molecules or cells can be composed for the formulation of a bioink [23]. A myriad of current reviews summarized the recent achievements in the field of bioinks [20,42,60–62]. According to these studies, natural biomaterial-based bioinks, especially alginate, gelatin and fibrin, are the most cited for vascular tissue engineering applications.

While designing a bioink, key features, namely, printability, stability, biology and rheology issues, should be seriously considered and balanced [20]. The viscosity, gelation and crosslinking capabilities are the basic characteristics to consider when selecting a bioink [19]. The deviation of the produced construct from the design depends on the bioink properties [27]. For example, an increased step in viscosity leads to an improved fidelity, but also an increased shear stress leads to cell damage and activation of misleading biophysical cues related to the ECM elasticity and pores' characteristics [20].

The fidelity of the 3D manufactured construct depends on the rapidness of transition to the solid state of the bioink after the deposition. After the ejection, the decrease of gelification time improves the structure's resolution [20]. Rheological and mechanical properties can be enhanced due to nanoparticles, with the inherent characteristic of drug delivery [63,64].

In Zhang et al.'s research, human umbilical vein smooth muscle cells and sodium alginate were combined, and vasculature conduits were printed through an extrusion printer, resulting in ECM formation and in increased proliferation rate [52]. Zigzag vascular tubes were fabricated through an inkjet-based bioprinter [65]. The viability of fibroblasts was at least 80% within 72 h of culture. In addition, the laser bioprinting technique improves the interplay between different types of cells and the formation of a vascular-like network [66].

The cell sources used in the bioprinting process could be classified into allogenic and autologous. Cardiomyocytes, human umbilical cord and embryonic stem cells were categorized in the first one, whereas adipose stem cell, skeletal stem cell, induced pluripotent stem cells (iPSCs) and bone marrow derived stem cells were put in the second category [67].

Maturation Methods of 3D Printed Vascular Grafts

The fabrication of vascular scaffolds is usually accompanied by post-curing methods for successful cell delivery. ECM proteins are frequently used to create a cell-supporting environment [68]. Jordahl et al. reported that extended 3D fibrillar fibronectin networks improved cell invasion and proliferation [68].

Efficient graft maturation favored by si RNA and poly-L-lysine (PLL) multilayers which deposited on polydopamine-coated substrates, thus a remarkable cell adhesion was noticed [69]. Low temperature plasma treatment can also be used for the treatment and maturation of polymeric scaffolds to obtain enhanced cell proliferation. More precisely, according to the research of Liu et al., nanofiber vascular scaffolds exhibited plasma treatment and the resulting hydrophilicity of these scaffolds effectively promoted vascular endothelial cell adhesion and proliferation [70]. Biocompatible photoabsorbers favor intricate scaffold maturation during the printing process. Grigoryan et al. used tartrazine, curcumin or anthocyaninc as photoabsorbers and improved the stereolithographic production of hydrogels, hence acquiring multilateral and functional vascular architectures [71]. Moreover, bioactive soft materials with enhanced biomimetic mechanical properties may result in graft maturation. Interestingly, in the Sun et al. study, magnesium ion incorporated into 3D printed polymer, where cell adhesion and proliferation were significantly promoted [72].

3. In Vivo Applications of 3D Bioprinting in CVD

The main aim of 3D bioprinting is to design functional tissues or parts of organs in situ for in vivo applications. The pivotal problem in terms of in vivo application is the compliance of cells and hydrogels, where cells need to precisely assemble themselves together exactly after printing, to achieve an adequate cell viability and vascularization of printed tissues. Cell–cell interaction for oxygen and nutrient interchange is mandatory to promote paracrine activity and homeostasis [73].

3.1. Cell Viability and Biocompatibility

Adequate cell viability is more than debatable in printed scaffolds due to high shear stresses on the cells delivered from extremely small diameter needle tips [62]. Cell viability decreases as the wall shear stress increases and the nozzle diameter of the deposition 3D bioprinting system decreases [74]. Overall, researchers should carefully select the cell density, the alginate concentration and dispensing pressure, and the coaxial nozzle size to obtain optimum cell viability on 3D bioprinted constructs [75].

Moreover, the estimation of cell viability is of paramount importance in order to decipher the interactions and stimulations between bioinks and cells, in a way that cells will satisfactorily adhere and survive [76]. Available methods for the evaluation of cell viability in 3D printed constructs are the common assays of trypan blue, release of LDH (lactate dehydrogenase), early apoptosis detection (Annexin V), Tetrazolium dye (MTT), study of DNA damage at the chromosome level (micronucleus assay) and other similar methods [77]. The optimum method to estimate cell viability, though, is fluorescent-based probes in the form of live/dead cells. Liu et al. utilized an improved in situ microscope method, where 3D constructs were split in order to investigate layer by layer the fluorescent number of cells and categorize live/dead cells [78].

Regarding in vivo studies, Bejleri et al. used bioprinted cardiac patches composed of native decellularized ECM and human cardiac progenitor cells (hCPCs). This specific combination of bioinks achieved cell viability of over approximately 75% [79]. Moreover, patches were retained on rat hearts and show vascularization over 14 days in vivo, indicating that the patches integrate well with the native myocardium inducing nutrient exchange with implanted cells.

Ong et al. suggested that in vivo implantation promoted vascularization of 3D bioprinted cardiac patches with engraftment into native rat myocardium [80]. In this study, multicellular cardiospheres consisted of human induced pluripotent stem cell derived cardiomyocytes (hiPSC-CMs), human adult ventricular cardiac fibroblasts (FBs) and human umbilical vein endothelial cells (ECs) assembled using a 3D bioprinter, and simultaneously the cell viability, in this patch, surpassed 90%.

Biocompatibility and circumvented cell cytotoxicity are mandatory in the field of 3D bioprinting materials as mentioned before. The in vivo study of Maxson et al. supports the potential use of a collagen-based bioink as an alternative for a tissue engineered heart valve implant [81]. Results of this study showed increased host cellularization potential, biocompatibility and biomechanical behavior results. The bioink was successfully printed with MSCs and showed remodeling.

3.2. Microarchitecture and Composition of 3D Construct Vascular Network

Three-dimensional bioprinting technology aims to combine different cell types and biomaterials heading to an enhanced cell repopulation within a 3D structure. An integrated vascular network is necessary to achieve cell viability in cardiovascular 3D printed tissues. Via that network, the influx and outflow of nutrients, metabolites and regulatory molecules are achieved. Large blood vessels ensure the flow in remote distances, whereas molecular diffusion occurs between capillaries and the surrounding tissue. In addition, the size of pores of 3D bioprinted constructs plays a major role for host cell recruitment. A pore size scaffolding >1 mm enables diffusion of nutrients until sufficient vascularization is achieved [82]. In the study of Shao et al., large scale constructs with mesoscale pore networks (100 μm to 1 mm) were successfully printed and the encapsulated vein endothelial cells were spread more efficiently compared to constructs without mesoscale pore networks [82]. In hydrogel-based scaffolding the preferable pore size of 1–150 μm provided structural support and adequate nutrient diffusion; specifically, in the study of

Zhang et al., 120–150 μm pore size resolution encouraged cells to gradually migrate into the microfibers to form a layer of confluent endothelium [83].

In the study of Maiullari et al. hydrogels and cells were printed layer by layer, thus emulating the native tissue architecture. Specifically, heterotypic human umbilical vein endothelial cells (HUVECs) and induced pluripotent cell-derived cardiomyocytes (iPSC-CMs) were transplanted hypodermically in mice and the bioprinted engineered tissue effectively merged with the host vasculature by providing enriched vascular networks [84].

Angiogenic factors play a pivotal role in the neovascularization of bioprinted cardiac tissues [85]. Notably, the tissue-engineered constructs need blood vessel development in the core. The Vascular Endothelial Growth Factor (VEGF) is used as such a regulator. VEGF regulates the vascular development and its therapeutic overexpression by the cells loaded into the construct. In this way, blood vessels sustainably grow directly into the core of the bio-engineered graft. Poldervaart et al. underlined the VEGF secretion from gelatin microparticles into the 3D constructs and the following vascularization was widely examined [85]. Further in vivo studies, regarding the effectiveness of 3D bioprinted materials, need to be implemented in order to overcome the challenge of VEGF overexpression with the intertwined side effect of vascular tumor growth (angioma) in the myocardium and other tissues [86].

3.3. Improved 3D Prined Grafts in Animal Models

Three-dimensional bioprinted cardiovascular grafts require robust control over a range of physical and mechanical properties that will enable bioink tailoring to a specific clinical application [62]. Overall, the greatest post-implantation challenge of 3D construct in cardiovascular tissue engineering is to maintain integrity and durability over time. Therefore, studies with animal models are necessary to improve the sustainability of 3D bioprinted cardiovascular grafts.

In the study of Melchiorri et al., 3D fabricated poly (propylene fumarate) PPF graft maintained mechanical properties, long-term mechanical support and physical parameters of graft (inner diameter and wall thickness) post six months of implantation in the venous system of the mice-selected animal model, while no thrombosis, aneurysm or stenosis were obtained [87]. In a rat animal model, 3D printed polyvinyl alcohol (PVA) mimicking 3D vascular grafts showed increased postoperative endothelialization during 30 days with significant decreased thrombogenesis [88]. Another study regarding a porcine animal model, utilized tissue engineered vascular graft (TEVG) with optimum anatomically fit and hemodynamic properties and adequate physical properties in a low-pressure venous system within one month [89].

4. Future Perspectives

New techniques to improve 3D bioprinting emerged due to intrinsic limitations of exogenous scaffolds or ECM-based materials [37]. Scaffold-free way of 3D bioprinting is one upcoming challenging approach to this endeavour. Tissue strands, cell sheets and spheroids, as a prefabricated block can be used for this purpose [90–92]. The "Kenzan" method is thought to be a pioneering method for bioprinting scaffold-free vascular grafts [93]. More precisely, spheroids are combined via micro-needles into contiguous structures. Thus, the achieved precision in a micron-level renders the method capable for tissue engineering purposes. In addition, the studies of Tseng et al. and Maina et al. introduce the magnetic 3D printing method [94,95]. Three-dimensional cellular blocks, which secrete their own ECM proteins, can be assembled with magnetic levitation. Bioinks of fibroblasts and smooth muscle cells are used for bioprinting cylindrical vessels 10 nm to 10 cm in length. Via this method, the scaffold degradation toxicity is remarkably eliminated.

Research on 3D printing and bioprinting has rapidly grown with the collaboration of various fields of expertise. Current breakthroughs in 3D bioprinting continue to broaden the spectrum of bioprinting methods and applications introducing nowadays 4D bioprinting which is expected to become the evolution of bioprinting and the next generation technology, as one more dimension of transformation over time is added [96]. In this way, dynamic 3D-patterned biological constructions could alter their microarchitecture by responding to external stimuli [97].

Merging 4D time controlled bioprinting features with innovative shape memory polymers (SMPs) paves the way to enhanced treatment in CVDs while maturation and functionalization of cells in 3D constructs alters over time [98]. Hence, the necessity of self-monitoring by regaining and maintaining their bioprinted properties over time may establish a remarkable evolution, especially in the field of personalized medicine.

5. Conclusions

In the realm of cardiovascular medicine, 3D bioprinting methodology leverages engineering-controlled viable biomimetic products to incorporate into clinically applicable cardiovascular grafts and tissues, heart patches, valves and other relative constructs. This review briefly summarizes the benefits and drawbacks of the 3D bioprinting method upon CVD treatment. To sum up, in order to treat a wide field of CVDs via the bioprinting method, a 3D bioprinted construct should meet the criteria of non-cytotoxicity, biodegradation, biocompatibility with preserved mechanical strength and structural integrity. Therefore, biomimicking the patient's tissue and thoroughly incorporating into surrounding tissues and organs, thus enhancing homeostasis and construct durability and viability. In conclusion, the 3D bioprinting method still has some limitations, but has mainly tangible improvements with in vivo application for clinical translation.

Funding: This research received no external funding.

Conflicts of Interest: The authors declare no conflict of interest.

References

1. WHO. Cardiovascular Diseases (CVDs). Available online: https://www.who.int/health-topics/cardiovascular-diseases#tab=tab_1 (accessed on 26 September 2021).
2. Mallis, P.; Kostakis, A.; Stavropoulos-Giokas, C.; Michalopoulos, E. Future Perspectives in Small-Diameter Vascular Graft Engineering. *Bioengineering* **2020**, *7*, 160. [CrossRef]
3. Gheorghe, A.; Griffiths, U.; Murphy, A.; Legido-Quigley, H.; Lamptey, P.; Perel, P. The economic burden of cardiovascular disease and hypertension in low- and middle-income countries: A systematic review. *BMC Public Health* **2018**, *18*, 975. [CrossRef]
4. Leal, J.; Luengo-Fernandez, R.; Gray, A.; Petersen, S.; Rayner, M. Economic burden of cardiovascular diseases in the enlarged European Union. *Eur. Heart J.* **2006**, *27*, 1610–1619. [CrossRef]
5. Tchantchaleishvili, V.; Schubmehl, H.; Swartz, M.F.; Hallinan, W.; Massey, H.T. Evolving strategies in the treatment of acute myocardial infarction-induced cardiogenic shock. *Ann. Cardiothorac. Surg.* **2014**, *3*, 606–611. [CrossRef] [PubMed]
6. Alrefai, M.T.; Murali, D.; Paul, A.; Ridwan, K.M.; Connell, J.M.; Shum-Tim, D. Cardiac tissue engineering and regeneration using cell-based therapy. *Stem Cells Cloning* **2015**, *8*, 81–101. [CrossRef] [PubMed]
7. Kim, J.Y.; Kim, J.B.; Jung, S.H.; Choo, S.J.; Chung, C.H.; Lee, J.W. Long-Term Outcomes of Homografts in the Aortic Valve and Root Position: A 20-Year Experience. *Korean J. Thorac. Cardiovasc. Surg.* **2016**, *49*, 258–263. [CrossRef]
8. Schmidt, C.E.; Baier, J.M. Acellular vascular tissues: Natural biomaterials for tissue repair and tissue engineering. *Biomaterials* **2000**, *21*, 2215–2231. [CrossRef]
9. Bouten, C.V.; Dankers, P.Y.; Driessen-Mol, A.; Pedron, S.; Brizard, A.M.; Baaijens, F.P. Substrates for cardiovascular tissue engineering. *Adv. Drug Deliv. Rev.* **2011**, *63*, 221–241. [CrossRef]
10. van Geldorp, M.W.; Eric Jamieson, W.R.; Kappetein, A.P.; Ye, J.; Fradet, G.J.; Eijkemans, M.J.; Grunkemeier, G.L.; Bogers, A.J.; Takkenberg, J.J. Patient outcome after aortic valve replacement with a mechanical or biological prosthesis: Weighing lifetime anticoagulant-related event risk against reoperation risk. *J. Thorac. Cardiovasc. Surg.* **2009**, *137*, 881–886. [CrossRef]
11. Wang, P.; Sun, Y.; Shi, X.; Shen, H.; Ning, H.; Liu, H. 3D printing of tissue engineering scaffolds: A focus on vascular regeneration. *Bio-Des. Manuf.* **2021**, *4*, 1–35. [CrossRef] [PubMed]
12. Murphy, S.V.; Atala, A. 3D bioprinting of tissues and organs. *Nat. Biotechnol.* **2014**, *32*, 773–785. [CrossRef]
13. Adhikari, J.; Roy, A.; Das, A.; Ghosh, M.; Thomas, S.; Sinha, A.; Kim, J.; Saha, P. Effects of Processing Parameters of 3D Bioprinting on the Cellular Activity of Bioinks. *Macromol. Biosci.* **2021**, *21*, e2000179. [CrossRef]
14. Zhang, B.; Gao, L.; Ma, L.; Luo, Y.; Yang, H.; Cui, Z. 3D Bioprinting: A Novel Avenue for Manufacturing Tissues and Organs. *Engineering* **2019**, *5*, 777–794. [CrossRef]
15. Mallis, P.; Michalopoulos, E.; Pantsios, P.; Kozaniti, F.; Deligianni, D.; Papapanagiotou, A.; Stavropoulos Giokas, C. Recellularization potential of small diameter vascular grafts derived from human umbilical artery. *Bio-Med Mater. Eng.* **2019**, *30*, 61–71. [CrossRef] [PubMed]

16. Zhu, J.; Marchant, R.E. Design properties of hydrogel tissue-engineering scaffolds. *Expert Rev. Med. Devices* **2011**, *8*, 607–626. [CrossRef] [PubMed]
17. Muschler, G.F.; Nakamoto, C.; Griffith, L.G. Engineering Principles of Clinical Cell-Based Tissue Engineering. *JBJS* **2004**, *86*, 1541–1558. [CrossRef]
18. França, F.S.; Garrido dos Santos, M.; Prestes, J.P.; Alcântara, B.; Borges, M.F.; Pranke, P. Bioprinting: A promising approach for tissue regeneration. *Bioprinting* **2021**, *22*, e00130. [CrossRef]
19. Malda, J.; Visser, J.; Melchels, F.P.; Jungst, T.; Hennink, W.E.; Dhert, W.J.; Groll, J.; Hutmacher, D.W. 25th anniversary article: Engineering hydrogels for biofabrication. *Adv. Mater.* **2013**, *25*, 5011–5028. [CrossRef]
20. van Kampen, K.A.; Scheuring, R.G.; Terpstra, M.L.; Levato, R.; Groll, J.; Malda, J.; Mota, C.; Moroni, L. Biofabrication: From Additive Manufacturing to Bioprinting. In *Encyclopedia of Tissue Engineering and Regenerative Medicine*; Reis, R.L., Ed.; Academic Press: Oxford, UK, 2019; pp. 41–55.
21. ASTM. Standard Terminology for Additive Manufacturing Technologies. In *Standard Terminology for Additive Manufacturing*; Astm International: West Conshohocken, PA, USA, 2013; p. F2792-12a. [CrossRef]
22. Bikas, H.; Stavropoulos, P.; Chryssolouris, G. Additive manufacturing methods and modelling approaches: A critical review. *Int. J. Adv. Manuf. Technol.* **2015**, *83*, 389–405. [CrossRef]
23. Moroni, L.; Boland, T.; Burdick, J.A.; De Maria, C.; Derby, B.; Forgacs, G.; Groll, J.; Li, Q.; Malda, J.; Mironov, V.A.; et al. Biofabrication: A Guide to Technology and Terminology. *Trends Biotechnol.* **2018**, *36*, 384–402. [CrossRef] [PubMed]
24. Sachs, E.M.; Haggerty, J.S.; Cima, M.J.; Williams, P.A. Three-Dimensional Printing Techniques. U.S. Patent 5,204,005, 20 April 1993.
25. Marti, P.; Lampus, F.; Benevento, D.; Setacci, C. Trends in use of 3D printing in vascular surgery: A survey. *Int. Angiol. J. Int. Union Angiol.* **2019**, *38*, 418–424. [CrossRef]
26. Geris, L.; Papantoniou, I. The Third Era of Tissue Engineering: Reversing the Innovation Drivers. *Tissue Eng. Part A* **2019**, *25*, 821–826. [CrossRef]
27. Kacarevic, Z.P.; Rider, P.M.; Alkildani, S.; Retnasingh, S.; Smeets, R.; Jung, O.; Ivanisevic, Z.; Barbeck, M. An Introduction to 3D Bioprinting: Possibilities, Challenges and Future Aspects. *Materials* **2018**, *11*, 2199. [CrossRef]
28. Sirry, M.S.; Zilla, P.; Franz, T. A Computational Study of Structural Designs for a Small-Diameter Composite Vascular Graft Promoting Tissue Regeneration. *Cardiovasc. Eng. Technol.* **2010**, *1*, 269–281. [CrossRef]
29. Zhang, S.; Vijayavenkataraman, S.; Lu, W.F.; Fuh, J.Y.H. A review on the use of computational methods to characterize, design, and optimize tissue engineering scaffolds, with a potential in 3D printing fabrication. *J. Biomed. Mater. Res. Part B Appl. Biomater.* **2019**, *107*, 1329–1351. [CrossRef]
30. Han, X.; Courseaus, J.; Khamassi, J.; Nottrodt, N.; Engelhardt, S.; Jacobsen, F.; Bierwisch, C.; Meyer, W.; Walter, T.; Weisser, J.; et al. Optimized vascular network by stereolithography for tissue engineered skin. *Int. J. bioprint.* **2018**, *4*, 134. [CrossRef]
31. Randles, A.; Frakes, D.H.; Leopold, J.A. Computational Fluid Dynamics and Additive Manufacturing to Diagnose and Treat Cardiovascular Disease. *Trends Biotechnol.* **2017**, *35*, 1049–1061. [CrossRef]
32. Groll, J.; Boland, T.; Blunk, T.; Burdick, J.A.; Cho, D.W.; Dalton, P.D.; Derby, B.; Forgacs, G.; Li, Q.; Mironov, V.A.; et al. Biofabrication: Reappraising the definition of an evolving field. *Biofabrication* **2016**, *8*, 013001. [CrossRef]
33. Moroni, L.; Burdick, J.A.; Highley, C.; Lee, S.J.; Morimoto, Y.; Takeuchi, S.; Yoo, J.J. Biofabrication strategies for 3D in vitro models and regenerative medicine. *Nat. Rev. Mater.* **2018**, *3*, 21–37. [CrossRef]
34. Lee, J.M.; Sing, S.L.; Zhou, M.; Yeong, W.Y. 3D bioprinting processes: A perspective on classification and terminology. *Int. J. Bioprint.* **2018**, *4*, 151. [CrossRef]
35. Chen, F.M.; Liu, X. Advancing biomaterials of human origin for tissue engineering. *Prog. Polym. Sci.* **2016**, *53*, 86–168. [CrossRef]
36. Williams, D.F. Challenges With the Development of Biomaterials for Sustainable Tissue Engineering. *Front. Bioeng. Biotechnol.* **2019**, *7*, 127. [CrossRef]
37. Norotte, C.; Marga, F.S.; Niklason, L.E.; Forgacs, G. Scaffold-free vascular tissue engineering using bioprinting. *Biomaterials* **2009**, *30*, 5910–5917. [CrossRef]
38. Chimene, D.; Kaunas, R.; Gaharwar, A.K. Hydrogel Bioink Reinforcement for Additive Manufacturing: A Focused Review of Emerging Strategies. *Adv. Mater.* **2020**, *32*, 1902026. [CrossRef]
39. Jang, J. 3D Bioprinting and In Vitro Cardiovascular Tissue Modeling. *Bioengineering* **2017**, *4*, 71. [CrossRef]
40. Barron, J.A.; Wu, P.; Ladouceur, H.D.; Ringeisen, B.R. Biological Laser Printing: A Novel Technique for Creating Heterogeneous 3 dimensional Cell Patterns. *Biomed. Microdevices* **2004**, *6*, 139–147. [CrossRef]
41. Rademakers, T.; Horvath, J.M.; van Blitterswijk, C.A.; LaPointe, V.L.S. Oxygen and nutrient delivery in tissue engineering: Approaches to graft vascularization. *J. Tissue Eng. Regen. Med.* **2019**, *13*, 1815–1829. [CrossRef]
42. Hann, S.Y.; Cui, H.; Esworthy, T.; Miao, S.; Zhou, X.; Lee, S.J.; Fisher, J.P.; Zhang, L.G. Recent advances in 3D printing: Vascular network for tissue and organ regeneration. *Transl. Res.* **2019**, *211*, 46–63. [CrossRef]
43. Cui, X.; Boland, T. Human microvasculature fabrication using thermal inkjet printing technology. *Biomaterials* **2009**, *30*, 6221–6227. [CrossRef]
44. Gao, Q.; He, Y.; Fu, J.Z.; Qiu, J.J.; Jin, Y.A. Fabrication of shape controllable alginate microparticles based on drop-on-demand jetting. *J. Sol-Gel Sci. Technol.* **2015**, *77*, 610–619. [CrossRef]
45. Gudapati, H.; Dey, M.; Ozbolat, I. A comprehensive review on droplet-based bioprinting: Past, present and future. *Biomaterials* **2016**, *102*, 20–42. [CrossRef]

46. Christensen, K.; Xu, C.; Chai, W.; Zhang, Z.; Fu, J.; Huang, Y. Freeform inkjet printing of cellular structures with bifurcations. *Biotechnol. Bioeng.* **2015**, *112*, 1047–1055. [CrossRef]
47. Xu, T.; Baicu, C.; Aho, M.; Zile, M.; Boland, T. Fabrication and characterization of bio-engineered cardiac pseudo tissues. *Biofabrication* **2009**, *1*, 035001. [CrossRef]
48. Jia, W.; Gungor-Ozkerim, P.S.; Zhang, Y.S.; Yue, K.; Zhu, K.; Liu, W.; Pi, Q.; Byambaa, B.; Dokmeci, M.R.; Shin, S.R.; et al. Direct 3D bioprinting of perfusable vascular constructs using a blend bioink. *Biomaterials* **2016**, *106*, 58–68. [CrossRef]
49. Li, Q.; Liu, C.; Wen, J.; Wu, Y.; Shan, Y.; Liao, J. The design, mechanism and biomedical application of self-healing hydrogels. *Chin. Chem. Lett.* **2017**, *28*, 1857–1874. [CrossRef]
50. Tabriz, A.G.; Hermida, M.A.; Leslie, N.R.; Shu, W. Three-dimensional bioprinting of complex cell laden alginate hydrogel structures. *Biofabrication* **2015**, *7*, 045012. [CrossRef]
51. Wenger, R.; Giraud, M.-N. 3D Printing Applied to Tissue Engineered Vascular Grafts. *Appl. Sci.* **2018**, *8*, 2631. [CrossRef]
52. Zhang, Y.; Yu, Y.; Akkouch, A.; Dababneh, A.; Dolati, F.; Ozbolat, I.T. In Vitro Study of Directly Bioprinted Perfusable Vasculature Conduits. *Biomater. Sci.* **2015**, *3*, 134–143. [CrossRef]
53. Mandrycky, C.; Wang, Z.; Kim, K.; Kim, D.H. 3D bioprinting for engineering complex tissues. *Biotechnol. Adv.* **2016**, *34*, 422–434. [CrossRef]
54. Elomaa, L.; Pan, C.C.; Shanjani, Y.; Malkovskiy, A.; Seppala, J.V.; Yang, Y. Three-dimensional fabrication of cell-laden biodegradable poly(ethylene glycol-co-depsipeptide) hydrogels by visible light stereolithography. *J. Mater. Chem. B* **2015**, *3*, 8348–8358. [CrossRef]
55. Gaebel, R.; Ma, N.; Liu, J.; Guan, J.; Koch, L.; Klopsch, C.; Gruene, M.; Toelk, A.; Wang, W.; Mark, P.; et al. Patterning human stem cells and endothelial cells with laser printing for cardiac regeneration. *Biomaterials* **2011**, *32*, 9218–9230. [CrossRef]
56. Zhu, W.; Qu, X.; Zhu, J.; Ma, X.; Patel, S.; Liu, J.; Wang, P.; Lai, C.S.; Gou, M.; Xu, Y.; et al. Direct 3D bioprinting of prevascularized tissue constructs with complex microarchitecture. *Biomaterials* **2017**, *124*, 106–115. [CrossRef]
57. Jana, S.; Lerman, A. Bioprinting a cardiac valve. *Biotechnol. Adv.* **2015**, *33*, 1503–1521. [CrossRef]
58. Koch, L.; Deiwick, A.; Franke, A.; Schwanke, K.; Haverich, A.; Zweigerdt, R.; Chichkov, B. Laser bioprinting of human induced pluripotent stem cells-the effect of printing and biomaterials on cell survival, pluripotency, and differentiation. *Biofabrication* **2018**, *10*, 035005. [CrossRef]
59. Shanjani, Y.; Pan, C.C.; Elomaa, L.; Yang, Y. A novel bioprinting method and system for forming hybrid tissue engineering constructs. *Biofabrication* **2015**, *7*, 045008. [CrossRef]
60. Gungor-Ozkerim, P.S.; Inci, I.; Zhang, Y.S.; Khademhosseini, A.; Dokmeci, M.R. Bioinks for 3D bioprinting: An overview. *Biomater. Sci.* **2018**, *6*, 915–946. [CrossRef]
61. Jang, J.; Park, J.Y.; Gao, G.; Cho, D.W. Biomaterials-based 3D cell printing for next-generation therapeutics and diagnostics. *Biomaterials* **2018**, *156*, 88–106. [CrossRef]
62. Holzl, K.; Lin, S.; Tytgat, L.; Van Vlierberghe, S.; Gu, L.; Ovsianikov, A. Bioink properties before, during and after 3D bioprinting. *Biofabrication* **2016**, *8*, 032002. [CrossRef] [PubMed]
63. Ahlfeld, T.; Cidonio, G.; Kilian, D.; Duin, S.; Akkineni, A.R.; Dawson, J.I.; Yang, S.; Lode, A.; Oreffo, R.O.C.; Gelinsky, M. Development of a clay based bioink for 3D cell printing for skeletal application. *Biofabrication* **2017**, *9*, 034103. [CrossRef] [PubMed]
64. Baumann, B.; Jungst, T.; Stichler, S.; Feineis, S.; Wiltschka, O.; Kuhlmann, M.; Linden, M.; Groll, J. Control of Nanoparticle Release Kinetics from 3D Printed Hydrogel Scaffolds. *Angew. Chem. Int. Ed.* **2017**, *56*, 4623–4628. [CrossRef] [PubMed]
65. Xu, C.; Chai, W.; Huang, Y.; Markwald, R.R. Scaffold-free inkjet printing of three-dimensional zigzag cellular tubes. *Biotechnol. Bioeng.* **2012**, *109*, 3152–3160. [CrossRef]
66. Gruene, M.; Pflaum, M.; Hess, C.; Diamantouros, S.; Schlie, S.; Deiwick, A.; Koch, L.; Wilhelmi, M.; Jockenhoevel, S.; Haverich, A.; et al. Laser printing of three-dimensional multicellular arrays for studies of cell-cell and cell-environment interactions. *Tissue Eng. Part C Methods* **2011**, *17*, 973–982. [CrossRef]
67. Chaudhuri, R.; Ramachandran, M.; Moharil, P.; Harumalani, M.; Jaiswal, A.K. Biomaterials and cells for cardiac tissue engineering: Current choices. *Mater. Sci. Eng. C* **2017**, *79*, 950–957. [CrossRef] [PubMed]
68. Jordahl, S.; Solorio, L.; Neale, D.B.; McDermott, S.; Jordahl, J.H.; Fox, A.; Dunlay, C.; Xiao, A.; Brown, M.; Wicha, M.; et al. Engineered Fibrillar Fibronectin Networks as Three-Dimensional Tissue Scaffolds. *Adv. Mater.* **2019**, *31*, e1904580. [CrossRef]
69. Hong, C.A.; Son, H.Y.; Nam, Y.S. Layer-by-layer siRNA/poly(L-lysine) Multilayers on Polydopamine-coated Surface for Efficient Cell Adhesion and Gene Silencing. *Sci. Rep.* **2018**, *8*, 7738. [CrossRef] [PubMed]
70. Liu, F.; Liao, X.; Liu, C.; Li, M.; Chen, Y.; Shao, W.; Weng, K.; Li, F.; Ou, K.; He, J. Poly(l-lactide-co-caprolactone)/tussah silk fibroin nanofiber vascular scaffolds with small diameter fabricated by core-spun electrospinning technology. *J. Mater. Sci.* **2020**, *55*, 7106–7119. [CrossRef]
71. Grigoryan, B.; Paulsen, S.J.; Corbett, D.C.; Sazer, D.W.; Fortin, C.L.; Zaita, A.J.; Greenfield, P.T.; Calafat, N.J.; Gounley, J.P.; Ta, A.H.; et al. Multivascular networks and functional intravascular topologies within biocompatible hydrogels. *Science* **2019**, *364*, 458–464. [CrossRef]
72. Sun, L.; Wang, M.; Chen, S.; Sun, B.; Guo, Y.; He, C.; Mo, X.; Zhu, B.; You, Z. Molecularly engineered metal-based bioactive soft materials—Neuroactive magnesium ion/polymer hybrids. *Acta Biomater.* **2019**, *85*, 310–319. [CrossRef]
73. Dawson, E.; Mapili, G.; Erickson, K.; Taqvi, S.; Roy, K. Biomaterials for stem cell differentiation. *Adv. Drug Deliv. Rev.* **2008**, *60*, 215–228. [CrossRef] [PubMed]

74. Nair, K.; Gandhi, M.; Khalil, S.; Yan, K.C.; Marcolongo, M.; Barbee, K.; Sun, W. Characterization of cell viability during bioprinting processes. *Biotechnol. J.* **2009**, *4*, 1168–1177. [CrossRef]
75. Yu, Y.; Zhang, Y.; Martin, J.A.; Ozbolat, I.T. Evaluation of cell viability and functionality in vessel-like bioprintable cell-laden tubular channels. *J. Biomech. Eng.* **2013**, *135*, 91011. [CrossRef]
76. Dubbin, K.; Hori, Y.; Lewis, K.K.; Heilshorn, S.C. Dual-Stage Crosslinking of a Gel-Phase Bioink Improves Cell Viability and Homogeneity for 3D Bioprinting. *Adv. Healthc. Mater.* **2016**, *5*, 2488–2492. [CrossRef] [PubMed]
77. Deo, K.A.; Singh, K.A.; Peak, C.W.; Alge, D.L.; Gaharwar, A.K. Bioprinting 101: Design, Fabrication, and Evaluation of Cell-Laden 3D Bioprinted Scaffolds. *Tissue Eng. Part A* **2020**, *26*, 318–338. [CrossRef] [PubMed]
78. Liu, N.; Huang, S.; Yao, B.; Xie, J.; Wu, X.; Fu, X. 3D bioprinting matrices with controlled pore structure and release function guide in vitro self-organization of sweat gland. *Sci. Rep.* **2016**, *6*, 34410. [CrossRef]
79. Bejleri, D.; Streeter, B.W.; Nachlas, A.L.Y.; Brown, M.E.; Gaetani, R.; Christman, K.L.; Davis, M.E. A Bioprinted Cardiac Patch Composed of Cardiac-Specific Extracellular Matrix and Progenitor Cells for Heart Repair. *Adv. Healthc. Mater.* **2018**, *7*, e1800672. [CrossRef]
80. Ong, C.S.; Fukunishi, T.; Zhang, H.; Huang, C.Y.; Nashed, A.; Blazeski, A.; DiSilvestre, D.; Vricella, L.; Conte, J.; Tung, L.; et al. Biomaterial-Free Three-Dimensional Bioprinting of Cardiac Tissue using Human Induced Pluripotent Stem Cell Derived Cardiomyocytes. *Sci. Rep.* **2017**, *7*, 4566. [CrossRef]
81. Maxson, E.L.; Young, M.D.; Noble, C.; Go, J.L.; Heidari, B.; Khorramirouz, R.; Morse, D.W.; Lerman, A. In vivo remodeling of a 3D-Bioprinted tissue engineered heart valve scaffold. *Bioprinting* **2019**, *16*, e00059. [CrossRef]
82. Shao, L.; Gao, Q.; Xie, C.; Fu, J.; Xiang, M.; Liu, Z.; Xiang, L.; He, Y. Sacrificial microgel-laden bioink-enabled 3D bioprinting of mesoscale pore networks. *Bio-Des. Manuf.* **2020**, *3*, 30–39. [CrossRef]
83. Zhang, Y.S.; Arneri, A.; Bersini, S.; Shin, S.R.; Zhu, K.; Goli-Malekabadi, Z.; Aleman, J.; Colosi, C.; Busignani, F.; Dell'Erba, V.; et al. Bioprinting 3D microfibrous scaffolds for engineering endothelialized myocardium and heart-on-a-chip. *Biomaterials* **2016**, *110*, 45–59. [CrossRef] [PubMed]
84. Maiullari, F.; Costantini, M.; Milan, M.; Pace, V.; Chirivì, M.; Maiullari, S.; Rainer, A.; Baci, D.; Marei, H.E.; Seliktar, D.; et al. A multi-cellular 3D bioprinting approach for vascularized heart tissue engineering based on HUVECs and iPSC-derived cardiomyocytes. *Sci. Rep.* **2018**, *8*, 13532. [CrossRef]
85. Poldervaart, M.T.; Gremmels, H.; van Deventer, K.; Fledderus, J.O.; Oner, F.C.; Verhaar, M.C.; Dhert, W.J.; Alblas, J. Prolonged presence of VEGF promotes vascularization in 3D bioprinted scaffolds with defined architecture. *J. Control. Release* **2014**, *184*, 58–66. [CrossRef]
86. Schwarz, E.R.; Speakman, M.T.; Patterson, M.; Hale, S.S.; Isner, J.M.; Kedes, L.H.; Kloner, R.A. Evaluation of the effects of intramyocardial injection of DNA expressing vascular endothelial growth factor (VEGF) in a myocardial infarction model in the rat—angiogenesis and angioma formation. *J. Am. Coll. Cardiol.* **2000**, *35*, 1323–1330. [CrossRef]
87. Melchiorri, A.J.; Hibino, N.; Best, C.A.; Yi, T.; Lee, Y.U.; Kraynak, C.A.; Kimerer, L.K.; Krieger, A.; Kim, P.; Breuer, C.K.; et al. 3D-Printed Biodegradable Polymeric Vascular Grafts. *Adv. Healthc. Mater.* **2016**, *5*, 319–325. [CrossRef]
88. Sohn, S.-H.; Kim, T.-H.; Kim, T.-S.; Min, T.-J.; Lee, J.-H.; Yoo, S.-M.; Kim, J.-W.; Lee, J.-E.; Kim, C.-H.; Park, S.-H.; et al. Evaluation of 3D Templated Synthetic Vascular Graft Compared with Standard Graft in a Rat Model: Potential Use as an Artificial Vascular Graft in Cardiovascular Disease. *Materials* **2021**, *14*, 1239. [CrossRef]
89. Yeung, E.; Inoue, T.; Matsushita, H.; Opfermann, J.; Mass, P.; Aslan, S.; Johnson, J.; Nelson, K.; Kim, B.; Olivieri, L.; et al. In Vivo implantation of 3-dimensional printed customized branched tissue engineered vascular graft in a porcine model. *J. Thorac. Cardiovasc. Surg.* **2020**, *159*, 1971–1981. [CrossRef]
90. Ovsianikov, A.; Khademhosseini, A.; Mironov, V. The Synergy of Scaffold-Based and Scaffold-Free Tissue Engineering Strategies. *Trends Biotechnol.* **2018**, *36*, 348–357. [CrossRef] [PubMed]
91. Akkouch, A.; Yu, Y.; Ozbolat, I.T.; Ozbolat, I.T. Microfabrication of scaffold-free tissue strands for three-dimensional tissue engineering. *Biofabrication* **2015**, *7*, 031002. [CrossRef]
92. Moldovan, L.; Barnard, A.; Gil, C.H.; Lin, Y.; Grant, M.B.; Yoder, M.C.; Prasain, N.; Moldovan, N.I. iPSC-Derived Vascular Cell Spheroids as Building Blocks for Scaffold-Free Biofabrication. *Biotechnol. J.* **2017**, *12*, 1700444. [CrossRef] [PubMed]
93. Moldovan, N.I.; Hibino, N.; Nakayama, K. Principles of the Kenzan Method for Robotic Cell Spheroid-Based Three-Dimensional Bioprinting. *Tissue Eng. Part B Rev.* **2017**, *23*, 237–244. [CrossRef] [PubMed]
94. Tseng, H.; Gage, J.A.; Haisler, W.L.; Neeley, S.K.; Shen, T.; Hebel, C.; Barthlow, H.G.; Wagoner, M.; Souza, G.R. A high-throughput in vitro ring assay for vasoactivity using magnetic 3D bioprinting. *Sci. Rep.* **2016**, *6*, 30640. [CrossRef] [PubMed]
95. Maina, R.M.; Barahona, M.J.; Finotti, M.; Lysyy, T.; Geibel, P.; D'Amico, F.; Mulligan, D.; Geibel, J.P. Generating vascular conduits: From tissue engineering to three-dimensional bioprinting. *Innov. Surg. Sci.* **2018**, *3*, 203–213. [CrossRef] [PubMed]
96. Javaid, M.; Haleem, A. 4D printing applications in medical field: A brief review. *Clin. Epidemiol. Glob. Health* **2019**, *7*, 317–321. [CrossRef]
97. Saska, S.; Pilatti, L.; Blay, A.; Shibli, J.A. Bioresorbable Polymers: Advanced Materials and 4D Printing for Tissue Engineering. *Polymers* **2021**, *13*, 563. [CrossRef]
98. Wan, Z.; Zhang, P.; Liu, Y.; Lv, L.; Zhou, Y. Four-dimensional bioprinting: Current developments and applications in bone tissue engineering. *Acta Biomater.* **2020**, *101*, 26–42. [CrossRef] [PubMed]

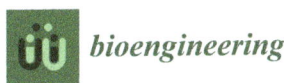

Review

Future Perspectives in Small-Diameter Vascular Graft Engineering

Panagiotis Mallis [1,*], Alkiviadis Kostakis [2], Catherine Stavropoulos-Giokas [1] and Efstathios Michalopoulos [1]

1. Hellenic Cord Blood Bank, Biomedical Research Foundation Academy of Athens, 4 Soranou Ephessiou Street, 115 27 Athens, Greece; cstavrop@bioacademy.gr (C.S.-G.); smichal@bioacademy.gr (E.M.)
2. Center of Experimental Surgery and Translational Research, Biomedical Research Foundation Academy of Athens, 4 Soranou Ephessiou Street, 115 27 Athens, Greece; akostakis@bioacademy.gr
* Correspondence: pmallis@bioacademy.gr; Tel.: +30-210-6597331; Fax: +30-210-6597345

Received: 25 October 2020; Accepted: 9 December 2020; Published: 10 December 2020

Abstract: The increased demands of small-diameter vascular grafts (SDVGs) globally has forced the scientific society to explore alternative strategies utilizing the tissue engineering approaches. Cardiovascular disease (CVD) comprises one of the most lethal groups of non-communicable disorders worldwide. It has been estimated that in Europe, the healthcare cost for the administration of CVD is more than 169 billion €. Common manifestations involve the narrowing or occlusion of blood vessels. The replacement of damaged vessels with autologous grafts represents one of the applied therapeutic approaches in CVD. However, significant drawbacks are accompanying the above procedure; therefore, the exploration of alternative vessel sources must be performed. Engineered SDVGs can be produced through the utilization of non-degradable/degradable and naturally derived materials. Decellularized vessels represent also an alternative valuable source for the development of SDVGs. In this review, a great number of SDVG engineering approaches will be highlighted. Importantly, the state-of-the-art methodologies, which are currently employed, will be comprehensively presented. A discussion summarizing the key marks and the future perspectives of SDVG engineering will be included in this review. Taking into consideration the increased number of patients with CVD, SDVG engineering may assist significantly in cardiovascular reconstructive surgery and, therefore, the overall improvement of patients' life.

Keywords: small-diameter vascular grafts; tissue engineering; cardiovascular disease; vascular reconstruction; bypass surgery; decellularization; human umbilical arteries; synthetic materials; 3D and 4D printing; thermoresponsive materials

1. Introduction

Small-diameter vascular grafts (SDVGs) with inner lumen diameter (d) less than 6 mm are required in vascular reconstructive surgery. Tissue engineering (TE) represents an emerging research field where the production of vascular grafts utilizing state-of-the-art manufacturing methods has gained great attention from the scientific society [1,2]. In contrast to large (d > 8 mm) and medium (d = 6–8 mm) diameter vascular grafts, which have currently been applied in a wide variety of vascular applications, such as carotid and aorta replacement, the production of SDVGs (d < 6 mm) requires further improvement [1–3]. Indeed, synthetic vascular grafts, derived from expanded polytetrafluoroethylene (ePTFE) and Dacron, serving as medium- or large-diameter vessel transplants, have shown interesting results in reconstructive surgery [4]. Long-term results of large diameter vascular grafts (LDVGs), e.g., when applied as aortoiliac substitutes, have exhibited good patency rates (90%) within the first year of implantation [2,5,6]. Additionally, medium-diameter vascular grafts, such as the carotid substitutes, are characterized by patency rates greater than 60% after the 1st year of implantation [2,7]. On the other hand, the proper production and use of small-diameter vascular grafts in reconstructive surgery are still under evaluation.

SDVGs are initially aimed to be used in coronary artery bypass grafting (CABG), issued by manifestations of cardiovascular disease (CVD). Regarding non-communicable diseases, CVD is the most leading cause of death globally [8,9]. CVD is a group of complex disorders, including peripheral arterial disease (PAD), coronary heart disease (CHD), cerebrovascular disease, and rheumatic heart disease [8,10]. It has been estimated that in the European Union (EU), CVD causes more than 3.9 million deaths, which accounts for 45% of all deaths each year [11]. Moreover, 11.3 million new cases of CVD are reported in the EU annually [12,13]. Furthermore, the United States is characterized by an increased percentage of CVD cases and deaths [14,15]. It is estimated that more than 400,000 CABG procedures are performed in the USA annually [14,16]. The CVD occurrence is mostly related to changes in dietary habits, reduced exercise, increased working time, depression, national health care deficiencies and the occurred financial crisis [17–20]. In terms of economic burden, it has been estimated that in Greece, the mean annual healthcare cost per patient is 5495 €, 4594 €, and 8693 € for CHD, CVD, and PAD, respectively [21]. Therefore, the proper development and clinical utilization of functional SDVGs is of paramount importance.

Nowadays, a great number of treatments can be effectively applied in CVD. These treatments may include the change of dietary–lifestyle habits or the application of pharmaceutical and surgical approaches. In the context of vascular surgery intervention, endovascular approaches such as angioplasty, atherectomy, and stent insertion can be performed. Additionally, vascular graft transplantation may be applied as an alternative option to replace or bypass the injured vessels.

To date, the gold standard procedure for CABG is the use of autologous vessels, such as the internal thoracic artery, radial artery, and saphenous vein [22]. Among them, the saphenous vein (SV) is the most widely used graft in SDVGs replacement [23–27]. The first use of saphenous vein in the clinical setting has been reported in 1951 by Kunlin and his colleagues [28]. The SV is characterized by greater patency rates (90% after the 1st year of implantation), compared to synthetic grafts (>60%, within the first year) [7,29,30]. However, significant drawbacks also accompany the use of autologous vessels. It is estimated that >30% of patients with CVD lack suitable vessels [1,31]. Moreover, in the case of the performance of second bypass surgery, the possibility of finding another suitable vessel decreases dramatically [32]. The latter can be performed within 10 years after the initial implantation, considering that the patency rate of autologous vessels (saphenous vein) after the 5 years is approximately less than 50% [2]. Moreover, biomechanical incompliance between arteries and veins can result in neointima formation, immune system activation, and finally graft failure and rejection [32].

Taking into account the above information regarding the use of SDVGs for bypass surgeries, alternative strategies for the development of vessel conduits must be evaluated and established. Tissue engineering may assist significantly to this issue by providing evidence and new ideas for the manufacturing of suitable SDVGs, which will be capable for cell homing, growth, and differentiation, and also characterized by improved in vitro and in vivo remodeling properties. In this review, we will highlight the state-of-the-art methodologies, while the future perspectives of SDVGs will be presented in detail.

2. Characteristics of Engineered SDVGs

The manufacturing of SDVGs with the TE methodologies has been improved significantly since the first attempts for production and application of synthetic vascular grafts used in bypass surgeries in the late 1980s [33]. Several years later, the first commercially available tissue-engineered vascular grafts (TEVGs) appeared, including Synergraft® (CryoLife, Inc., Kennesaw, GA, USA), Artegraft® (LeMaitre Vascular, Inc., Burlington, MA, USA), Procol® (LeMaitre Vascular, Inc., Burligton, MA, USA), and Cryovein® (CryoLife, Inc., Kennesaw, GA, USA) [34]. The majority of these grafts have received approval from the Food and Drug Administration (FDA) and the European Medicinal Agency (EMA) for human applications.

The proper design of the vascular grafts ensures successful cell seeding at the pre- and post-implantation stage. Cellular populations may positively influence the vessel graft functionality [35]. The most applied cellular populations are the endothelial cells (ECs) and vascular smooth muscle cells (VSMCs) [36]. ECs are located in the internal layer of the vascular wall, known as tunica intima, forming the endothelium [37]. The endothelium has unique anti-thrombogenic properties, avoiding the platelet aggregations and clots formation [38]. VSMCs are responsible for vasoconstriction and vasodilation, located in the media layer of the vessel wall, which is known as tunica media [39]. Dependent on microenvironment stimuli, the ECs can elevate the levels of endothelial nitric oxide synthetase (eNOS), leading to NO production, which downstream induces the VSMCs-dependent vasodilation [38]. Importantly, VSMCs also support the vascular remodeling and regeneration with the production of extracellular matrix (ECM) proteins such as collagen and elastin [39]. Besides, the beneficial effects of the cellular populations may occur to the vascular graft, their successfully seeding and proliferation may require long-term cultivation periods. Additionally, the isolation and expansion of specialized cellular populations from patients with CVD is a demanding challenge [40]. To date, there is a tendency for developing readily available acellular vascular scaffolds with improved anti-thrombogenic properties [41–44]. Indeed, these pioneering studies are focusing on the fabrication of a negatively charged synthetic surface in order to avoid red blood cells and platelet aggregation. In this way, the SDVGs must satisfy certain design criteria to be clinically available [45]. Specifically, SDVGs must have similar biomechanical properties (burst pressure, high-stress deformation, and suture strength) with the substituted vessels to avoid aneurysm and neointima development [46]. In addition, regardless of the vascular graft material, engineered vessels must be non-cytotoxic and support cell growth [45]. Engineered SDVGs must be characterized by specific ultrastructure, ensuring the cell seeding, proliferation, and differentiation [2]. Finally, the engineered SDVGs must not be immunogenic, and also must be characterized by in vivo remodeling and regeneration properties [2].

Nowadays, a wide variety of manufacturing techniques for SDVGs such as the use of synthetic polymers, decellularized natural matrices, bioprinting, and 4D printing have been developed, although the majority of them require further evaluation and optimization.

3. TEVGs Derived from Synthetic Polymers

Manufactured TEVGs from polymer materials have been widely used in vascular reconstructive surgery in the last years [47,48]. The use of synthetic polymers has brought a new era in surgery, decreasing the time needed for vessel conduit manufacturing. Vascular grafts produced from synthetic materials can be manufactured with state-of-the-art tissue engineering methods, including tissue engineering by self-assembly (TESA), electrospinning, and bioprinting. Among them, bioprinting has gained great attention from the scientific society due to the production of high-quality tissue engineering vascular scaffolds. The manufactured scaffolds (acellular or cellularized conduits) can be implanted in the patient to replace the damaged vessels (Figure 1). Synthetic conduits can be divided into non-degradable, degradable polymers, and biopolymers. Each category is characterized by specific characteristics, which will be further explored in this review article.

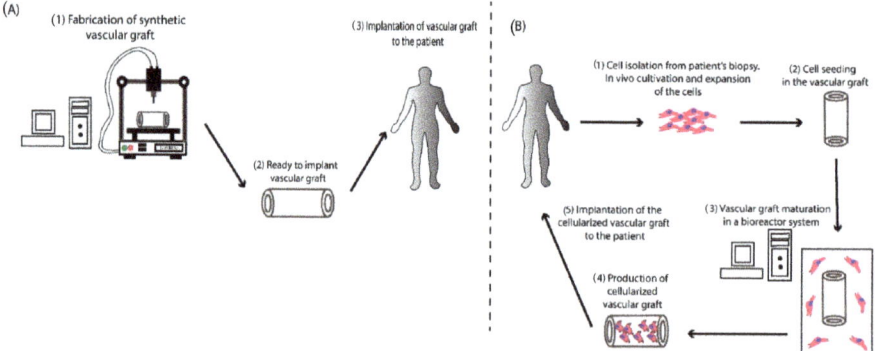

Figure 1. Development and implantation of engineered small-diameter vascular grafts (SDVGs). (**A**) The first approach comprises the production of acellular SDVG derived from polymer materials using the state-of-art bioprinting approach. Then, the manufactured SDVG can be implanted immediately into the patient. In this approach, the patient's body will serve as a bioreactor for the recellularization of the implanted vascular graft. However, some major disadvantages, including the time period needed for the proper cellularization or the impaired functionality of the produced vascular grafts, maybe existed. (**B**) The second approach comprises the combination of cellular populations with the polymer derived SDVGs. In this approach, the cells can be isolated from the patient's tissue biopsy, in vitro expanded, and seeded onto the SDVG. Finally, the engineered SDVG can be implanted back to the patient. The advantage of this approach is the production of compatible SDVGs with the patients, avoiding in this way any potential adverse reactions.

3.1. Non-Degradable Polymers

Non-degradable polymers were among the first materials used as a source for the production of vascular grafts that have been employed in bypass surgeries (Table 1). Historically, the first attempt for the production of ePTFE material has been performed by Robert Gore in 1969 [4]. Several years later, Campbell et al. reported promising results regarding the use of ePTFE vascular grafts in 15 patients as a femoropopliteal bypass graft [49]. In 1986, Weinberg and Bell [33] developed the first tissue-engineered blood vessel substitute through culturing of bovine ECs, VSMCs, and fibroblasts to a Dacron derived conduit. Since then, a great effort by the research teams has been performed establishing new strategies to obtain functional TEVGs. EPTFE, Dacron, and polyurethanes are the most used materials for the production of non-degradable vessel conduits [48]. Compared to autologous vessels, synthetic non-degradable conduits are characterized by a lower percentage of patency rates when used as SDVGs [50]. To date, Dacron is preferred to be used as a material for the production of vessel conduits due to improved biomechanical properties [48,51]. However, both of them exhibit significant adverse reactions. Specifically, a generalized immune response toward the polymers is exerted mostly by macrophages and T cells [52,53]. This could lead to lumen occlusion, which may be treated with new cardiovascular reconstructive surgery. Moreover, most of these grafts lack arginine-glycine-aspartic acid (RGD) binding sites in order to promote cell adhesion [54]. In this direction, several alternative strategies have been employed such as the chemical modification or pre-coating of the polymer materials toward favoring the cell adhesion. Indeed, the addition of P15 peptide, pre-coating with fibronectin, or cross-linked RGD binding sites have been suggested as alternative strategies for improving ECs and VSMCs seeding on polymer scaffolds [55]. A number of research groups have performed pre-coating of polymer vascular grafts with fibroblast growth factor (FGF), vascular endothelial growth factor (VEGF), and epidermal growth factor (EGF), improving in this way the ECs, VSMCs, and fibroblasts mobilization, seeding, and proliferation onto the produced graft [56–58]. Randone et al. [59] reported the efficient production of VEGF pre-coated ePTFE vascular grafts. The results of this study showed increased ECs proliferation and endothelium formation in VEGF pre-coated grafts compared to non-pre-coated vascular grafts. In addition, Randone et al. reported that the microporous structure of ePTFE was ideal for ECs seeding, thus grafts with high porosity (>90 μm) may have better endothelialization outcomes [59]. It is known that VEGF exerts chemoattractant and mitogenic abilities on ECs. In this way, the ECs can be attracted by the VEGF pre-coated graft [60]. During ECs proliferation, a significant amount of growth factors are released, which can further regulate the function of vessel resident cellular populations, such as the VSMCs and the fibroblasts [61].

Another important issue that should be addressed is the possibility of thrombus formation. Typically, the polymer acellular vascular grafts are preferred mostly due to the short manufacturing time that is needed. On the other hand, the absence of an organized endothelium could result in increased platelet aggregation and thrombus formation [62,63]. This series of events can cause serious adverse events to the patients that might be even life-threatening. A possible solution to this issue could be the production of polymers with anti-thrombogenic surface or polymers with the substantial release of anti-thrombogenic molecules. Hoshi et al. [64] have reported the successful production of heparin-modified ePTFE vascular grafts. Moreover, Hoshi et al. managed to develop an easily implemented approach, including the covalent link of heparin to the inner side of the ePTFE grafts, to produce vascular grafts with anti-thrombogenic properties [64]. The produced graft inhibited successfully the platelet adhesion; however, a minor negative effect in endothelial cell function was evident. Furthermore, heparin-modified ePTFE vascular grafts were characterized by the high stability of their modified surface area, which was retained for a long time period (28 days) [64]. Moreover, it should be noted that non-degradable polymers are characterized by specific biomechanical properties. Mismatch of tubular compliance may exist in vascular grafts derived from non-degradable polymers. This phenomenon is mostly occurred due to the pre-existing differences in elasticity between the TEVG and the native artery. It is known that small diameter arteries, which are characterized by specific mechanical properties, can absorb energy (pulsatile energy) during the vasoconstriction, which is further released during vasodilation, contributing to the pulsatile blood flow. In this way, a vascular graft, which is characterized by a stiffer behavior than the native ones, can diminish the pulsatile energy by 60%. This compliance mismatch between the two vessels can lead to intima hyperplasia, immune system overactivation, and final graft failure.

Table 1. Representative applications of tissue-engineered vascular grafts (TEVGs) derived from non-degradable polymers.

Material Composition	Application	Comments	Research Team
Dacron	In vitro	Successful EC seeding in Dacron vessel conduits using either collagen-coated Dacron or fibronectin-coating ePTFE grafts	Sugawara et al. [65]
Dacron	In vitro	Coating of Dacron-based vascular graft with polyurethane. Increased porosity to the inner surface of the graft. Improved cell attachment properties	Phaneuf et al. [66]
ePTFE	Implantation in rabbits	ePTFE grafts were used as carotid artery interposition grafts, Good patency rate after 28 days of implantation, Successful endothelialization	Hytonen et al. [67]
ePTFE	In vitro	Isolation of porcine ECs from jungular vein Successful endothelialization of ePTFE grafts Development of a bio-hybrid scaffold for vascular applications	Mall et al. [68]
ePTFE	Implantation in distal infrarenal aorta of rabbits	Development of ammonia plasma modified grafts Improved endothelialization of graft's inner surface.	Sipehia et al. [69]

Table 1. Cont.

Material Composition	Application	Comments	Research Team
ePTFE	In vitro and in vivo evaluation	Development of polyurethane/polyurethane film Improved antiplatelet properties Lower hemolysis and no cytotoxicity (in vitro) Better biocompatibility, no occlusion, and successful endothelialization	Zhang et al. [70]
Dacron and ePTFE	In vitro	Immobilization of heparin, collagen, laminin, prostaglandin E1 (PGE1) Reduction of fibrinogen adsorption, and platelets deposition. Improved biocompatibility properties of both grafts	Chandy et al. [71]
Dacron and ePTFE	Implantation in mongrel dogs	Thrombus formation was reported 3 and 4 weeks postoperatively in ePTFE grafts. Patency rate of ePTFE grafts drop from 66% (3 weeks) to 33% (4 weeks) Patency rate of Dacron grafts changed from 55% (3 weeks) to 44% (4 weeks) ECs seeded grafts presented better patency rates and no graft occlusion due to thrombus formation. All animals received antiplatelet treatment	Hikro et al. [72]

3.2. Degradable Polymers

Degradable polymers can be used as an alternative strategy for the production of SDVGs (Table 2). These materials can be substantially degraded, forming a proper ECM [47]. Hydrolysis of the ester bonds of the scaffolds and the metabolism of polymers into H_2O and CO_2 comprises the main degradation mechanism. The most known degradable materials are the poly (lactide-co-glycolide) (PLGA), polyglycolic acid (PGA), poly-lactic acid (PLA), poly-l-lactic acid (PLLA), polyglycerol sebacate (PGS), and polycaprolactone (PC) [47,48]. The above materials have been extensively used for the production of TEVGs with large and medium lumen diameter. Currently, these polymers have been proposed as starting materials for the production of SDVGs, while their efficient in vivo application is still under evaluation. Each material is characterized by unique properties. Indeed, the molecular structure, the polymerization transition temperature, and biomechanical behavior are some of the different properties that may exist among the materials [73]. For instance, PGA is characterized by rapid degradation time, which affects its biomechanical properties [47,48]. For this purpose, the degradation time can be controlled through polymerization with other materials such as PLA. PGS, another material that is used for the fabrication of TEVGs, can be fully degraded within 30 days [47,48]. PLA is a material whose complete degradation may last over years [2]. This material is characterized by a stiffer behavior than the PGA and also by improved endothelialization and patency rates. PCL is a hydrophobic material with long-term degradation time and, due to this, can sustain better initial biomechanical properties [47,48]. The first report regarding the biocompatibility and biodegradability of the polymer materials was performed in 1966 by Kulkarni and his colleagues [74]. Specifically, it was shown that PLA does not bear any cytotoxic factors and could be used in various applications, such as the production of surgical implants, without causing any tissue reaction.

Degradable polymers represent a valuable source for the production of acellular large, medium, and small diameter vessel conduits, reducing the manufacturing time even more. On the other hand, significant adverse reactions have been reported regarding their use. One major drawback is the lack of RGD-binding motifs, leading to ineffective cell seeding and proliferation [75]. As a consequence, organized endothelium cannot be formed, which can result in platelet aggregation, clot formation, and lumen occlusion [43]. For this purpose, several research groups are evaluating novel strategies for the efficient endothelialization of the luminal surface of the polymer-derived vascular grafts [2,47,48,76]. Previous strategies including chemical modifications and lumen surface pre-coating have also been employed to scaffolds derived from degradable polymers to improve further their functionality. Wang et al. [77] managed to develop an SDVG using a combination of PCL and gelatin. In addition, surface modification with heparin was also performed [77]. The produced vascular conduits were implanted in rats as an abdominal artery graft and remained patent for 12 weeks [77]. These grafts were proven capable of efficient recellularization by ECs. In the same way, Quint et al. [78] used a PGA vascular graft as a scaffold for in vitro recellularization with aortic SMCs. Then, these grafts were placed in a pulsatile bioreactor system for 10 weeks followed by decellularization [78]. The occurred acellular vascular graft was reseeded with ECs and endothelial progenitor cells (EPCs) in order to avoid thrombus formation. Finally, the vascular conduit was implanted to a porcine model as a common carotid artery interposition graft and remained for 30 days [78]. The results of this study showed the efficient production of a personalized vascular graft, which has retained its ability for in vivo remodeling [78]. To date, a small number of clinical trials with degradable SDVGs have been performed (Table 2). Specifically, Lawson et al. [79] developed PGA-based SDVGs that were initially repopulated with VSMCs in a bioreactor setting. Then, pulsatile cyclic distension for 8 weeks, was applied to the SDVGs, followed by decellurization procedure. The occurred acellular SDVGs were applied as an arteriovenous graft in 60 patients (divided into two studies). In both studies, the average primary patency rate was 58% and 23%, after 6 and 12 months, respectively [79]. No aneurysm formation or immune response against the SDVGs was observed in all patients. In total, 4 patients died from end-stage renal disease (ESRD) manifestations rather than vascular graft complications. Moreover, histological analysis in SDVGs segments after 16 weeks of implantation showed infiltration by CD68$^+$ monocytic cells, SMA$^+$ VSMCs, and CD31$^+$ ECs [79]. On the contrary, no T or B cells were evident in the histological analysis. The above outcome is quite promising, widening in this way the clinical feasibility of degradable SDVGs.

Table 2. Representative applications of TEVGs derived from degradable polymers.

Material Composition	Application	Comments	Research Team
PCL	In vitro	Production of electrospun PCL SDVGs Modified surface with polyethyleneimine and heparin Prolonged anticoagulant action of the modified SDVGs Mild inflammation reaction (when implanted subcutaneously) May be characterized by great long-term patency. Future plan, implantation to animal models	Wang et al. [77]
PCL	Implantation in sheep	Thrombosis formation in the control group Good patency rate of PCL SDVGs (50% after 1st year of implantation)	Antonova et al. [80]
PCL	Implantation in mice	Acellular electrospun PCL-derived vascular grafts implanted as a carotid interposition graft Successful recellularization by host's cells Complete endothelium formation within 28 days	Chan et al. [81]
PCL and PU	In vitro	Production of endothelialized SDVGs Good Biomechanical properties No significant differences in hemocompatibility between non-endothelialized and endonthelialized SDVGs	Mervado—Pagan et al. [82]
PGS	In vitro	Minimal platelet adhesion in the produced vascular graft No cytotoxicity to erythrocytes	Liu et al. [83] Motlagh et al. [84]

Table 2. Cont.

Material Composition	Application	Comments	Research Team
PLA	Implantation into rats	Antithrombogenic properties of MSCs Successful in vivo remodeling process Improved patency rate and no graft occlusion in BM-MSCs seeded vascular grafts	Hashi et al. [85]
PGA	In vitro	PGA derived vascular graft, seeded with VSMCs Maturation in a pulsatile flow bioreactor for 8 weeks Improved biomechanical properties (burst pressure 2150 mmHg)	Niklason et al. [86]
PGA	Implantation in baboons, canine	Implantation in baboons as arteriovenous conduits Implantation in canines as coronary artery interposition graft. Recellularization of PGA vascular graft with ECs. No aneurysm formation was reported Good patency rate in the majority of the vascular grafts after 1, 3, and 6 months in both animal models. Recellularization with host's VSMCs and ECs	Dahl et al. [87]
PGA	In vitro and in vivo	Recellularization of PGA vascular graft with ECs and maturation in a pulsatile flow bioreactor ECs and induced pluripotent stem cells (iPSCs) in vascular tissue engineering	Gui and Niklason. [88]
PGA	Human Use	Recellularization of PGA vascular grafts with human ECs obtained from cadaveric donors Implanted in 59 patients as arteriovenous graft Improved patency rate compared to ePTFE grafts.	Lawson et al. [79]

3.3. Biopolymers

Besides the use of non-degradable and degradable vascular grafts, conduits based on natural matrices and proteins have also been proposed as an alternative solution (Table 3) [1]. These proteins can be used as the structural basis for the development of SDVGs, providing an appealing 3D microenvironment with proper binding sites for the cellular populations [47,48]. Several methods have been proposed to properly produce biopolymer-based SDVGs, including electrospinning, freeze-drying, and mold casting.

Collagen and its isoforms are the most abundant proteins that can be easily isolated, manipulated, and used for scaffold production, including also the engineered SDVGs. Habermehl et al. [89] optimized the procedure for collagen isolation from rat tails, and since then, a wide number of applications, where this structural protein is the main player, have been reported [90–93]. Until now, 28 different collagen types have been reported [94]. The collagen structure is composed of a repeated triple helix of proline (X) and hydroxyproline (Y). Based on the triple helix organization, collagen can be distinguished into a) fibrils (including types I-V and XI), networks (including types IV-X), and filaments (including type VI) [94]. Among them, collagen I is the most abundant type in mammalians, composed of two $\alpha_1(I)$ and one $\alpha_2(I)$ chains. Collagen type I offers a great number of integrin-binding sites, which can control the cell adhesion, differentiation, and overall cellular behavior. Different types of collagen-based scaffolds have been used in tissue engineering applications [91]. Collagen scaffolds combined with hydroxyapatite have been used in orthopedic applications, inducing bone and cartilage regeneration [95,96]. Moreover, collagen has been proposed as a drug delivery system (DDS) to release pro-angiogenic factors for wound healing applications and as a natural coating of vascular grafts [97,98]. However, collagen is characterized by low mechanical properties and increased thrombogenicity [99,100]. For this purpose, cross-linking with fixative agents such as glutaldeyhyde has been proposed [101,102]. Nevertheless, the improvement in mechanical properties, severe cytotoxicity are accompanied most of the time due to the crosslinking agent that was applied [103]. Alternative crosslinking methods have also been utilized such as photo-crosslinking or the use of carbodiimide [104–106]. Moreover, collagen-based SDVGs combined with fibronectin or elastin fibers have shown promising results regarding the biomechanical and anti-thrombogenic properties. Another promising biomaterial for SDVGs fabrication is the silk fibroin [107,108]. Fibroin is derived from Bombyx mori (silkworm) and is composed of β-sheet crystal and semicrystalline regions occurred after the removal of sericin [109,110]. Sericin is a highly antigenic protein, which covers the silk fibers [111]. Additionally, fibroin has anti-thrombogenic properties and can be degraded over time, therefore, could be a valuable source for the production of SDVGs [112]. Enomoto et al. [113] managed to develop a fibroin-based SDVG whose patency was compared with ePTFE vessel conduits. In this study, the developed conduits (d = 1.5 mm, l = 10 mm) were implanted as abdominal aorta interposition grafts in male Sprague-Dawley rats for a time period of 72 weeks [113]. Fibroin based SDVGs remained patent (85%) over 64 weeks, whereas ePTFE grafts were patent (48%) for 32 weeks [113]. In addition, an increased number of SMCs and ECs was observed in fibroin-based SDVGs compared to ePTFE grafts, reflecting in this way the impaired overall functionality of the latter.

To date, fibrin, which can be obtained from peripheral blood, comprises a biomaterial that can be applied in SDVG engineering [114,115]. Fibrin is produced through the cleavage of fibrinogen [115]. Fibrinogen (MW: 340 kDa), a glycoprotein that is abundant in plasma, contains three pairs of polypeptide chains, the Aα, Bβ, and γ, which are connected with 29 disulfide bonds [115]. Upon stimulation, thrombin cleaves the fibrinopeptides A and B, between Arg-Gly residues [115,116]. The remained (α, β, γ)$_2$ can be polymerized with other fibrin molecules, resulting in the production of fibrin final form. Due to that, fibrin can be produced from patients' blood, without causing any negative adverse reactions to the recipient [115,116]. Fibrin is a rich source of growth factors, cytokines, and chemokines, such as Tumor Necrosis Factor-A (TNF-A), Vascular Endothelial Growth Factor (VEGF), Fibroblast Growth Factor (FGF), Platelet-Derived Growth Factor AA (PDGF-AA), Interleukin 1A (IL-1A), IL-1B, IL-2, IL-6, IL-8, TNF-Receptor type-1 associated Death domain protein (TRADD), CC-motif chemokine receptor 1, etc. [117,118]. Recently, platelet-rich plasma or fibrin gel have been employed in a series of regenerative medicine applications such as skin wound healing and dystrophic recessive epidermolysis bullosa [119,120]. Except for the patient's own blood, fibrin can be produced from other sources like the umbilical cord blood (UCB). Rebulla et al. [121] initially optimized the PRP and fibrin production from UCB units that did not meet the criteria for cryopreservation. In addition, our group suggested a protocol for the efficient production of PRP and fibrin from low volume CBU units [118]. The development of allogeneic fibrin holds significant advantages such as the avoidance of repeating blood sampling, especially from severe conditioned or elderly individuals, low immunogenicity of the obtained fibrin, and absence of allergic reaction [118].

Recently, fibrin has been employed in vascular tissue engineering. In the beginning, fibrin was used as a coating in collagen-based vascular grafts [122]. To date, the research society is performing a significant effort to produce fibrin-based vascular grafts [123,124]. Most of the time, a pulsatile bioreactor system is required for the proper maturation of the developed vascular grafts. Moreover, approaches where ECs and SMCs are utilized in fibrin-based vascular grafts, have been proposed [36]. Swartz et al. [125] used recellularized fibrin-based vascular grafts as implants in a sheep model. Specifically, these grafts were implanted in the jugular veins for a time period of 15 weeks. Histological analysis of the grafts showed the successful in vivo remodeling, where collagen and elastin depositions were evident [125]. However, the fibrin-based vascular grafts were characterized by impaired biomechanical properties. Indeed, the average burst pressure of fibrin-based vascular grafts was 543 ± 77 mmHg, which is very low to withstand the physiological burst pressures of blood flow [125]. A recent study from Yang et al. [126] showed that the mechanical properties of these vessel conduits can be improved with the addition of PCL, resulting in the production of a hybrid graft (fibrin-PCL vascular graft). In this study, electrospun PCL/fibrin vascular grafts were developed, followed by evaluation of mechanical properties, cytotoxic effects, and in vivo biocompatibility [126]. The burst pressure of these hybrid vascular grafts was 1811 ± 101 mmHg, which is similar to native blood vessels (2000 mmHg). Furthermore, no cytotoxic effects or in vivo immune response were reported, in this study [126].

The production of vascular grafts made of chitosan has also been reported [127]. Chitosan is a linear polysaccharide that is closely related to sulfated glycosaminoglycans (sGAGs) [128]. Chitosan is a natural material that is derived from the shell of shrimps and crabs and has been used extensively in a wide range of tissue engineering applications [128]. Specifically, chitosan has been used for the production of hydrogels, DDS, coatings, and also in wound healing applications [128]. In addition, chitosan can be combined with degradable polymers such as PCL and PLA for scaffold fabrication [129]. Moreover, chitosan has mild antibacterial properties, which are beneficial for in vivo applications [130]. Recently, the use of chitosan has been proposed for the development of SDVGs. In the context of vascular graft production, the electrospinning technology can be utilized to produce conduits with wide pore distribution, high porosity, and adequate microenvironment for cell adhesion and proliferation. Wang et al. [127] reported the development of a PCL/chitosan (PCL/Ch) hybrid-based SDVG with anti-thrombogenic and anti-bacterial properties. For the scaffold fabrication, the electrospinning technology was utilized [127]. The results of this study showed that the PCL/Ch hybrid-based SDVGs have similar anti-thrombogenic properties as the heparin-coated vessel conduits, while the bacterial killing ratios were 64% for *S. aureus* and 73% *E. coli* [127]. Yao et al. [129] also developed electrospun PCL/Ch SDVGs, which were further combined with heparin and referred as Hep-PC/Ch grafts. These grafts were further implanted as aortic replacements in male Sprague-Dawley rats. Their functionality was compared with PCL/Ch vascular grafts (without heparin immobilization). After 4 weeks of implantation in rats, the PCL/Ch explants were characterized by thrombus formation, while no thrombus formation was observed to Hep-PCL/Ch grafts [129]. Furthermore, Hep-PCL/Ch grafts were characterized by good patency rate and successful endothelialization as were indicated by SEM analysis [129]. Taking into consideration the above data, chitosan is a material that can be used in combination with degradable polymers to produce functional SDVGs.

Table 3. Representative applications of TEVGs derived from biopolymers.

Material Composition	Application	Comments	Research Team
Fibrin	In vitro	Combination of human dermal fibroblasts with vascular graft derived from fibrin gel Successful cell migration and collagen deposition Low biomechanical properties (burst pressure 543 mmHg)	Huyhn et al. [131]
Fibrin	In vivo	Fabrication of fibrin-based vascular graft Maturation of the graft in a pulsatile flow-stretch bioreactor Significant biomechanical properties (burst pressure 3164 ± 342 mmHg) corresponded to 99.8% of the reported value of human internal mammary artery Implantation as arteriovenous graft in olive male baboons The majority of the grafts remained patent for 6 months. Successful repopulation by host's cells	Syedain et al. [132]
Fibrin	In vivo	Production of fibrin-based vascular grafts, seeded with ovine dermal fibroblasts. Implantation of the grafts as pulmonary artery replacements in Dorset lamps Implanted grafts were characterized by physiological strength and stiffness, complete lumen endothelialization, and repopulation by SMCs The lamps exhibited somatic growth and normal physiological function for nearly one year.	Syedain et al. [133]

Table 3. Cont.

Material Composition	Application	Comments	Research Team
Fibrin, collagen, collagen-fibrin	In vitro	Collagen and collagen fibrin vascular grafts share common biomechanical properties Fibrin-based vascular grafts are characterized by lower biomechanical properties than the above grafts SMCs proliferated equally in all vascular scaffolds	Cummings et al. [134]
Hyaluronan	In vitro	Addition of sodium ascorbate to hyaluronan-based vascular grafts Improvement in SMC proliferation and cell viability. Well organized ECM and good biomechanical properties	Arrigoni et al. [135]
Silk	In vivo (Implantation into Sprague-Dawley rats as abdominal aorta graft)	Better patency rate after 1 year of implantation, compared to ePTFE graft ECs and SMCs proliferation into the grafts within a short time after the implantation Good ECM organization and in vivo remodeling properties (inner and media layer) Observation of vasa vasorum	Enomoto et al. [113]
Silk	In vivo	Silk-based vascular grafts have equal mechanical properties as the rat abdominal aorta. Low platelet adhesion High proliferation potential of silk-based vascular grafts seeded with HUVECs and SMCs Vascular remodeling after implantation experiments in rats	Lovett et al. [136]
Collagen	In vivo	Development of collagen-based vascular grafts with burst pressure 1313 mmHg Endothelialization of collagen tubes after implantation in femoral artery of rats	Li et al. [137]
Chitosan	In vitro	Development of chitosan (2% w/v) vascular graft Burst pressure over 4000 mmHg Successful seeding with VSMCs obtained from rabbit aorta	Zhang et al. [138]

3.4. Hybrid Polymers

The proper combination of synthetic and natural polymers could produce functional engineered SDVGs. These conduits combine the beneficial features of both materials and are characterized by improved biomechanical, anti-thrombogenic, anti-bacterial, and cell adhesion properties [139]. Furthermore, hybrid vascular grafts can be combined with key specific growth factors such as TGF-β1, VEGF, EGF, HGF, etc., which can be accumulated in the vascular wall [129,140,141]. These growth factors can be spatially released from there, affecting in this way several cellular functions including cell migration and growth [142]. To date, there is an increasing number of research teams, which are focusing on the production of hybrid vessel conduits (Table 4). Tillman et al. [143] produced a PCL/collagen vascular graft, with improved biomechanical properties. The PCL/collagen conduits served as the aorta and iliac artery interposition grafts in rabbits and remained for a time period of 1 month [143]. These hybrid grafts were free of any aneurism or thrombus formation, while Doppler ultrasound showed good patency (85%) of the grafts. Histological analysis of the explants revealed the absence of inflammation, thus completely lacking any infiltrating immune cell [143]. Wise et al. [144] produced PCL/elastin vascular grafts, where parameters such as ECs adhesion and proliferation, blood biocompatibility, burst pressure, and in vivo functionality were assessed [144]. Specifically, these grafts were able to be recellularize both in vitro and in vivo with the ECs. The burst pressure of the grafts was 1500 ± 150 mmHg; however, it was less than the minimum burst pressure that was evident in human native blood vessels (1700 mmHg). Similar good patency and cell infiltration results of hybrid acellular vascular grafts have been reported in the literature [144–147].

In addition to these fabrication strategies, the use of cellularized hybrid vascular grafts may provide better outcomes regarding the mechanical properties and overall patency [34]. Thomas and Nair [148] developed a vascular graft, which was composed of gelatin/vinyl acetate copolymers, utilizing the electrospinning method. The composed vascular grafts were successfully recellularized with murine SMCs, followed by maturation with a pulsatile bioreactor system [148]. The pulsatile forces, generated by the bioreactor, effectively stimulated the SMCs migration, proliferation, and gene and protein expression [149].

Table 4. Representative applications of TEVGs derived from hybrid materials.

Material Composition	Application	Comments	Research Team
PCL/collagen	In vivo	Development of hybrid scaffold with electrospinning method. Applied in aortoiliac bypass in rabbits, the graft remained for 1 month. Minimal cellular infiltration in the implanted vascular graft. Patency rate was 87.5% after 1 month of implantation	Tillman et al. [143]
PET/PU/PCL	In vitro and In vivo	Development of an electrospun triad-hybrid graft with an inner diameter of 5 mm. Burst pressure over 1689 mmHg Successful cell seeding and proliferation as it was indicated by the MTT assay Moderate immune reaction was observed after subcutaneous implantation in rats	Jirofti et al. [150]
PU/PET	In vitro	Development of PU/PET SDVGs with the electrospinning method Comparable biomechanical properties with native veins and arteries	Khodadoust et al. [151]
PU/PCL	In vitro	No cytotoxic PU/PCL vascular graft Successful seeded and proliferation of fibroblasts and ECs, as it was indicated by the MTT assay Confirmation of cell adhesion by SEM analysis	Nguyen et al. [152]
Gelatin/vinyl acetate	In vitro	Development of electrospun gelatin/vinyl acetate vascular grafts/ SMCs are used for seeding applications. Well organized ECM, accompanied by good biomechanical properties	Thomas and Nair et al. [148]
PCL and PU/collagen	In vivo	Electrospun PCL and PU/collagen vascular grafts were implanted as femoral artery interposition grafts in canines The grafts remained patent for 8 weeks Infiltration by ECs resulted in endothelium development	Lu et al. [153]
PCL/elastin	In vivo	Electrospun PCL/elastin vascular grafts were implanted as carotid arteries bypass grafts in rabbits The hybrid vascular graft was characterized by good biomechanical properties (tensile strength and Young's Elastic Modulus) Low platelet attachment Preservation of biomechanical properties after implantation	Wise et al. [144]

The overwhelming increase of new CVD cases each year is leading to the exploration of alternative sources for the production of engineered SDVGs. Most of these approaches, including non-degradable, degradable, and biopolymer grafts, are requiring extended evaluation, while their proper fabrication could last over 28 days [2,34]. Toward these shortcomings, the hybrid-based TEVGs may pose a reliable approach, reducing the manufacturing time and thus producing SDVGs with improved properties.

However, more research is needed to be performed in order for the hybrid SDVGs to be readily used by clinicians in cardiovascular reconstructive surgery.

4. Decellularized Vascular Grafts

In the last decade, the application of the decellularization method for the production of vascular grafts has gained significant attention from the scientific society [154]. Decellularization aims to remove completely the cellular material from the tissue while preserving the ultrastructure of ECM. Depending on the tissue source, different decellularization approaches may be applied to produce effectively an acellular matrix [154,155]. Until now, decellularization has been applied successfully to a great number of organs and tissues, including lung, liver, kidney, heart, cartilage, etc.

4.1. Decellularization as a Method for the Production of Vascular Grafts

To achieve the production of an acellular matrix, different decellularization protocols may be used. Mostly, the decellularization protocols include physical, chemical, enzymatic, or a combination of those methods to acquire the best outcome [154–156]. The initial step of the decellularization approach is cell destruction through the solubilization of the cytoplasmic membrane and DNA fragmentation. Then, the cellular and nuclear debris must be completely removed from the tissue's ECM. Excessive removal of decellularization solutions also is an important step of the process to limit the possibility of any cytotoxic effects [154–156]. The final step of the decellularization procedure is the sterilization of the produced scaffold.

Sterilization can be achieved either by immersion of the scaffold into antibiotic solutions or by applying physical methods such as UV and γ-irradiation [155,156].

The increased global demand for vascular grafts led the researchers to evaluate further the decellularization approach for the production of vessel conduits [36]. Large- and small-diameter vascular grafts have been decellularized with the application of different decellularization approaches. Mostly, a proper combination of the decellularization approaches, such as snap freezing, use of ionic and non-ionic detergents, trypsin addition, and mechanical agitation or sonication, have been utilized [154,156]. Among them, the use of chemical compounds in combination with physical methods, is the most effective and safe for producing acellular vascular grafts. The most used detergents for the decellularization procedure are sodium dodecyl sulfate (SDS), sodium deoxycholate (SD), Triton X-100, Triton X-200, 3-[(3-Cholamidopropyl)dimethylammonio]-1- propane sulfonate (CHAPS), and Ethylenediaminetetraacetic acid (EDTA) [156]. Additionally, in the literature, the combination of hypotonic and hypertonic treatments, with enzymatic digestion, has been also reported for the efficient production of acellular SDVGs [154–156].

Taking into consideration the above data, vascular grafts and especially SDVGs can be derived from various sources such as animals (porcine or sheep) or cadaver donors, effectively decellularized, and immediately used (Figure 2). However, significant drawbacks are accompanying the above proposal. In the past, a great effort regarding the use of animal-derived TEVGs in human applications was performed [157]. Despite the complete removal of cellular and nuclear materials from the vessel's ECM, animal-derived vascular grafts can induce an extended immune response due to the presence of alpha-gal-epitope (Galalpha1-3Galbeta1-(3)4GlcNAc-R) [158]. This epitope is abundant in non-primates and New World monkeys and synthesized by the alpha1,3galactosyltransferase (alpha1,3 GT) [158–160]. On the other hand, humans, apes, and Old World monkeys produce anti-Gal antibodies, which are representing 1% of the circulating immunoglobulins [158–160]. In this way, human recipients when receiving animal-derived vascular grafts, exert significant immune response against the aforementioned grafts, which finally leads to graft rejection. Nowadays, much effort has been focused on the cleavage of a-gal epitope or the production of transgenic animals (without the presence of a-gal epitope), although more research must be performed toward this direction [161,162]. Recently, genome editing with CRISPR-Cas9 may assist in this field [163]. Cadaver donors may constitute an alternative source, for obtaining SDVGs. Based on organ donation statistics, only 3 in 1000 people find suitable organs and more than 112,000 people are waiting for organ transplantation [164]. Furthermore, the bioethics rules must be modified in order to allow organ transplantation and especially vessel transplantation. The production of vascular grafts with the decellularization approach may be a promising approach, thus increasing the number of available transplantable vessels.

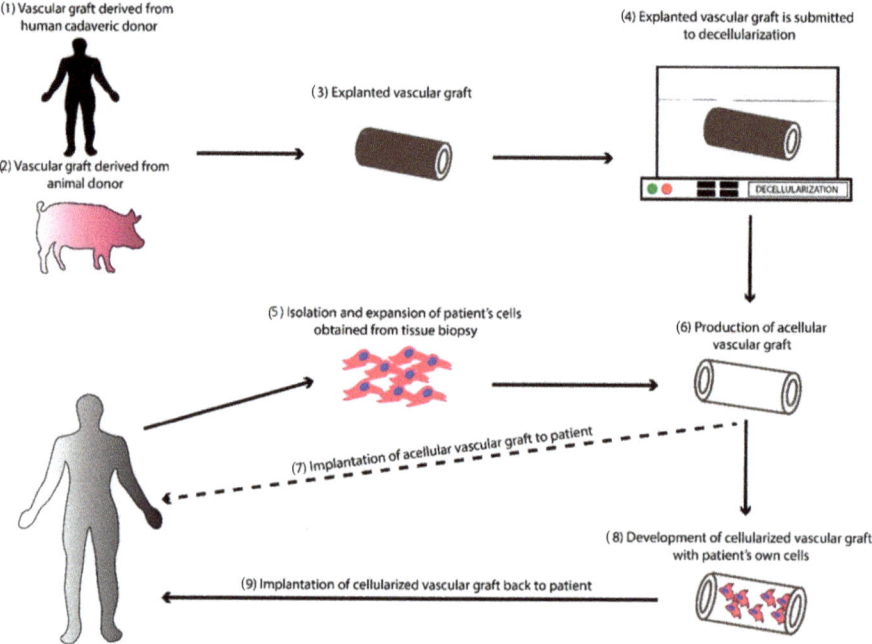

Figure 2. Production of SDVGs with the decellularization approach. Initially, vascular grafts can be obtained either from human cadaveric or animal donor. Then, the obtained SDVG is submitted to decellularization to remove the residual cellular population. The produced acellular vascular graft can be either implanted back to the patient or to submitted in recellularization with the patient's own cells. The cellular populations can be isolated and expanded from the patient's tissue biopsy. When cells reached the desired cell number, they can be used for the recellularization of the acellular vascular graft. Finally, the produced cellularized SDVG can be implanted in the patient. The whole procedure can be performed under good manufacturing practice (GMP) conditions.

4.2. Establishment of the Decellularization Approach

The production of a completely acellular scaffold is a demanding process; however, most of the time a small quantity of residual cellular and nuclear materials are evident. Different decellularization methods are characterized by variable results, indicating that the majority of them cannot produce a completely acellular scaffold. The presence of the cellular components could induce an immune response and hyperacute reaction by the host upon implantation [165,166]. This could lead to unfavorable adverse reactions, resulting in graft occlusion, calcification, and rejection, with the majority of them to be life-threatening for the recipients. Globally, several researchers have tried to validate the decellularization approach in different tissues and organs, leading them to several criteria for the establishment of the successful decellularization approach. Among them, Gilbert et al., Crapo et al., and Badylak et al. have performed the most valuable work, proposing the following criteria [154,156,167].

- <50 ng/double-stranded (ds) DNA/mg ECM dry weight
- <200 bp DNA fragmented length

- Lack of visible nuclear materials, either with 4′,6-diamidino-2-Phenylindole (DAPI) or hematoxylin and eosin (H&E)

Except for the above-mentioned criteria, the total amount of DNA including single-stranded (ss) and ds, should also be quantified and taken into account. DNA quantification can be performed photometrically, or with the use of different commercial kits such as the Picogreen Assay. Indeed, there are numerous studies where Picogreen assay is the optimum method for the quantification of the DNA in decellularized matrices [168–171]. However, the PicoGreen assay can detect only the ds DNA, while the ss DNA cannot be quantified. On the other hand, the spectrophotometric quantification of DNA by measuring the ratio of absorbance 260 nm/280 nm, may provide more data regarding the presence of the total DNA in the acellular scaffold [172]. It is known that either ss or ds DNA can induce the host's immune reaction, and the accurate DNA quantification is of major importance. Furthermore, the remaining DNA in the scaffolds can be evaluated through the performance of gel electrophoresis [172]. Typically, the DNA samples can be loaded onto 1–2% *w/v* agarose gels and observed under UV light. The absence of dense DNA bands or bands with less than 200 bp DNA confirms further the successful decellularization [172].

The last criterion involves the observation of the tissue sections for any possible nuclear material either with H&E or DAPI [154,156]. H&E is the first-line histological stain that is performed in order to properly evaluate the success of the decellularization approach. The absence of black stain in the histological samples indicates the loss of nuclear material. Besides H&E, more specific stains can be applied for the determination of decellularization. Masson's trichrome (MT), which stains collagen (blue), muscle cells (red), and nuclear materials (black), can be used for the evaluation of the presence or absence of SMCs. Except for the content of the cellular population, this stain can indicate the proper preservation of the collagen fibers in the acellular scaffold. In the same way, Elastic van Gieson (EVG) can stain simultaneously the elastic/collagen fibers and nuclear material [154,156].

Nevertheless, the production of a completely acellular scaffold is optimum, and the preservation of key ECM features such as the orientation of collagen and elastin fibers are also important. The microarchitecture structure of tissues and organs can determine the decellularization approach, which will be selected. Complex tissues, where the orientation of collagen and elastin determine eventually their biomechanical properties, can be decellularized with the use of non-enzymatic approaches [173–175]. It has been shown that trypsin can damage significantly the collagen fibers of a tissue, affecting in this way possibly the graft's biomechanical properties and cell-binding sites. A balance between the proper elimination of cellular components in combination with the minimum effect in ECM key proteins must be found when a decellularization protocol is applied.

4.3. Decellularized Animal-Derived SDVGs

The first attempt for establishing a decellularization protocol was performed in 1966, several years before the attempts of Weinberg and Bell for the manufacturing of synthetic polymer vascular graft [33]. Rosenberg et al. [176] applied for the first time an enzymatic decellularization protocol in bovine carotid arteries. The produced acellular vascular grafts were implanted in 16 patients as femoropopliteal and iliofemoral bypass grafts. The implanted grafts withstood the blood flow pressure; however, graft occlusion was reported during a time period of 2 years postoperatively [176]. Since then, new decellularization approaches have been found and validated in a wide range of tissues and organs including the vessels such as the aorta, carotid, and coronary arteries (Table 5) [177–180]. The first decellularized vascular grafts were derived from bovine vessels and ureters, which further became commercially available as Artegraft®, Solcograft®, ProCol® (LeMaitre Vascular, Inc., Burligton, MA, USA), etc. [2,181]. Today, several companies are focused on the production of decellularized vascular conduits based on the bovine vessels. However, the presence of a-gal is a significant limitation, and in order to overcome this issue, crosslinking with fixative agents such as glutaraldehyde is performed [103]. A significant drawback to this approach is the cytotoxicity mediated by the fixative agents, resulting in minimum applicability of those grafts [103]. However, modern fixative agents such as carbodiimide with low or no cytotoxicity have been applied [106]. Another significant drawback of the crosslinked decellularized bovine blood vessels is the lack of in vivo remodeling properties, which makes them unavailable for applications in pediatric patients [182]. Additionally, it has been reported that decellularized animal-derived blood vessels are characterized by similar patency rates as synthetic vascular grafts [36].

Recently, the use of small intestine submucosa (SIS) has been also proposed for the production of large and small TEVGs [183]. Typically, SIS can be derived either from the porcine or ovine origin [184]. Decellularization can efficiently be applied in SIS, and then the produced material can be folded in a tubular mandrel to produce a vascular graft [184]. Moreover, crosslinking with fixative agents such as glutaraldehyde has been reported as an important step in the manufacturing process [185]. These grafts currently have been evaluated for their functionality in animal models, showing good patency rates [36]. Moreover, the patency rates were superior or equal to ePTFE grafts and native ovine artery [36].

Table 5. Summary of representative studies toward decellularized animal-derived vascular grafts.

Material Composition	Application	Comments	Research Team
Bovine carotid artery	In vitro	Decellularization of bovine carotid arteries with 1% w/v SD, 1% w/v CHAPS, 1% v/v Triton X-100 or 0.1% SDS Successful decellularization of carotid arteries Preservation of ECM structure Good biomechanical properties	Daugs et al. [186]
Ovine carotid artery	In vitro	Decellularization of carotid arteries with 1% w/v SDS, 0.05% v/v Trypsin, 0.02% EDTA Histological analysis with H&E, Masson's Trichrome, and Verhoeff van Gieson revealed the preservation of ECM structure. Successful seeding and recellularization with MSCs	Mancuso et al. [187]
SIS	In vivo	Development of a vascular graft utilizing porcine SIS Implantation as a carotid artery interposition graft Functional comparison with autogenous saphenous vein No aneurism formation was found in both grafts. Equal patency rates between the two grafts	Sandusky et al. [188]
Bovine ureter	In vivo	Decellularized based on a patented process Comparison between ePTFE and decellularized bovine ureter. Applied as arteriovenous conduits Enrolled 60 patients No significant advantage of decellularized bovine ureter compared to ePTFE as AVF	Chemla and Morsy [189]
Bovine mesenteric vein	In vivo	Bovine mesenteric vein (MVB) evaluated as a vascular graft in hemodialysis Compared with ePTFE vascular graft Better patency rates of MVB than ePTFE graft (12 months was 35.6% for MVB versus 28.4% synthetic grafts. At 24 months, secondary patency was 60.3% MVB, 42.9% synthetic) Superior vascular graft compared to ePTFE grafts	Katzman et al. [190]
Canine carotid artery	In vivo	Decellularization of canine carotid arteries with 0.5% v/v Triton X-100, 0.05% v/v ammonium hydroxide Seeded with bone marrow MSCs derived from canine animal models Seeded grafts were implanted as carotid arteries interposition grafts Comparable suture retention strength between native and decellularized carotid arteries Successful in vivo remodeling after implantation, collagen and elastin production	Cho et al. [191]

Nowadays, the cost production of synthetic vascular grafts has been reduced and, considering the above data, their application is more preferable [36]. On the other hand, due to the increased demand for SDVGs, alternative sources must be explored in order to cardiovascular surgeons to have more available options.

4.4. Decellularized Human-Derived SDVGs

The first human blood vessel conduits served as transplants in reconstructive surgery were derived from human cadaver femoral veins. Indeed, human femoral arteries were submitted to decellularization to produce acellular vascular conduits [192]. These grafts were used initially as arteriovenous fistulas (AVF) allografts [193]. Furthermore, these grafts were commercialized under the name Synergraft® (CryoLife, Inc., Kennesaw, GA, USA) [34]. Decellularized iliac vein is another human vascular graft that has been proposed for vascular reconstruction applications [194]. Moreover, this graft was recellularized with the patient's cells such as ECs and SMCs and then was applied in a 10-year-old female patient with extrahepatic vein obstruction [195]. Before the cell seeding, the graft was evaluated for the presence of cell/nuclear materials and HLA class I and II genes. The operation was performed at Sahlgrenska University Hospital in Gothenburg, Sweden, and the outcomes were published in 2012 [195]. After 1 year of implantation, the graft was occluded, explanted, and a new vein graft was used. Finally, the patient responded well, no anti-endothelial cell antibodies were detected, and there was no need for receiving any immunosuppressive agents [195]. In this direction, human umbilical vessels may be an alternative source for the production of SDVGs [196]. The human umbilical cord (hUC) contains approximately two arteries and one vein, which are mediating in gas exchange and nutrient supply through the fetomaternal circulation [197]. The human umbilical arteries (hUAs) are responsible for the transportation of non-oxygenated blood from the fetus to the mother, while the human umbilical vein (hUV) performs exactly the opposite process [198]. The HUAs and hUVs are characterized by three layers, the inner (tunica intima), the media (tunica media), and the external layer (tunica adventitia). In addition, the hUAs and hUV are vessels without branches and their entire length can be varied and is dependent on hUCs length [197]. The length of a typical hUC is 20–60 cm and is characterized by an average number of 40 helical turns. In addition, hUAs are characterized by specific protrusions located in the tunica intima, throughout the entire vessels, which are known as "Hoboken valves" [199]. These valves prevent successfully the reflux of the non-oxygenated blood back to the fetus. Both vessels can easily and non-invasively be isolated from the hUC after gestation. Typically, in the case of using the human umbilical blood vessels, signed informed consent from the mothers must be obtained [196]. The informed consent should fulfill the requirements of the National law, regarding cord tissue donation and also should be in accordance with the Helsinki declaration.

HUV has been applied as a vascular bypass graft since 1974, followed by commercialization, which was known as Biograft® [200,201]. Several years later, the outcome of the use of Biograft® was evaluated. Specifically, a comprehensive evaluation of the use of hUV as a femoropopliteal bypass graft, a study involved 133 operations and a 5-year follow up, was performed [202]. In this study, it was shown that 6% of the patients died within 30 days after the implantation. The majority of the complications in patients were evident within the first 3 months postoperatively. The mean patency rate was 65% and 50% within the first and fifth year, respectively. No infection of the graft was reported in the current study [202]. The obtained results of the current study indicated that the stabilized hUV could potentially be used as a source for SDVG production. Currently, the gold standard autologous graft for coronary artery bypass surgeries is the SV [203]. However, other blood vessel sources have been evaluated such as the cephalic artery, stabilized hUV, and ePTFE grafts (Table 6). Among them, the hUV seems to share better patency and biocompatibility properties compared to the cephalic and ePTFE vessel conduits [204]. Indeed, a randomized clinical trial has shown that the patency rate of ePTFE was 40% within the first year of implantation, while stabilized hUV was 75% for the same time period [204]. Moreover, SV and stabilized hUV seems to share similar patency rates. Although the results were quite promising, the hUV was stopped to be used as a vessel substitute due to significant drawbacks [204]. HUV is more difficult to be applied technically than SV or synthetic conduits. Moreover, hUV may lack elasticity, making it more fragile [200–202,204,205]. In addition, the crosslinking reagents used for its stabilization like glutaraldehyde could induce severe cytotoxicity. Another drawback that is accompanied by the use of the crosslinking agents is the lack of in vivo remodeling properties, which make it less available for pediatric patients [204].

Taking into consideration the above data, the use of hUAs as possible vascular conduits should be also evaluated. Kerdjoudj et al. [206,207] used for the first time the human umbilical artery as potential small-diameter vascular grafts. Initially, this approach involved the deposition of a synthetic polyelectrolyte film in hUAs in order to avoid the platelet adhesion and eventually the thrombus formation [206,207]. In this study, the hUAs were enzymatically de-endothelialized and treated with poly(styrene sulfonate)/poly(allylamine hydrochloride) (PSS/PAH) to develop multilayers of polyelectrolyte film. This negative polyelectrolyte film can exert key anti-thrombogenic properties, avoiding in this way the platelet accumulation and thrombus formation in the lumen surface of the vessels. Then, these grafts were implanted as carotid interposition grafts in rabbits and remained for a time period of 3 months [206]. The results of this study were impressive, indicating the long-term patency (over 12 weeks) of the hUAs treated with PSS/PAH film. Furthermore, successful cell invasion of $PECAM^+$ ECs and $\alpha\text{-}SMA^+$ SMCs was evident in tunica intima and media, respectively [206]. Minimum intimal hyperplasia was reported in these grafts, which were mainly exerted through collagen production from SMCs [206]. Several months later, Gui et al. [208] evaluated a novel decellularization protocol in hUAs. In this study, a series of important experiments were performed, obtaining valuable information regarding the utilization of the hUAs as SDVGs [208]. Furthermore, the decellularized hUAs were implanted as abdominal interposition grafts in nude rats. After 8 weeks of implantation, thrombus formation was observed in the vascular grafts. Despite this drawback, decellularized hUAs sustained the blood flow and finally, the vessel did not rupture [208]. Several years later, the comprehensive proteomic analysis combined with histological data in native and decellularized hUAs was performed [209]. Until now, several researchers have evaluated the possibility of using the hUAs as transplants [206–211]. In 2020, our group showed that the decellularized hUA can be successfully vitrified and stored at −196 °C over a long time period [172]. Specifically, vitrified (decellularized) hUAs retained the ECM structure after 2 years of storage in liquid nitrogen. Furthermore, the vitrified grafts were used for common carotid bypass grafting in porcine animal models and remained for a time period of 1 month. Although the occurrence of platelet aggregation and thrombus formation was observed, vitrified hUAs were successfully in vivo remodeled [172]. The grafts were recellularized by the host's VSMCs, and due to the blood flow stress-strain forces, increased production of elastin fibers was occurred [172]. By the time that this publication is prepared, another work from our group is focused on the biomechanical and proteomic characteristics of the decellularized hUAs [212]. The proteomic results have been deposited to the ProteomeXchange Consortium with the dataset identifier PXD020187 (https://www.ebi.ac.uk/pride/) and are currently publicly available. In this study, a rapid decellularization protocol was effectively applied in hUAs. No cellular or nuclear remnants were evident, while at the same time the proteomic and biomechanical analysis showed the preservation of key ECM structural proteins and mechanical characteristics of the hUAs, respectively [212].

HUAs may represent a better source for the development of SDVGs compared to hUVs. However, extended validation experiments to better determine the stability and functionality of these grafts should be performed. The future goal will be the successful recellularization with ECs/VSMCs and implantation to large animal models for longer time periods to acquire more valuable data regarding the possible application of hUAs as SDVGs.

Table 6. Summary of representative studies toward decellularized human-derived vascular grafts.

Material Composition	Application	Comments	Research Team
Cadaveric femoral vein	In vivo (large-scale clinical trial)	Commercially available decellularized human femoral vein (Synergraft®) Applied as allograft for Hemodialysis Comparison between Synergraft®, Cryovein and ePTFE grafts Impaired patency rate of human allografts compared to ePTFE grafts Aneurism formation observed in human allografts Human allografts cost 5 times more than ePTFE grafts Ethical concerns	Madden et al. [213]
Iliac vein	In vivo (Proof of concept study)	Decellularization of iliac vein with 1% v/v Triton X-100, 1% v/v tri-n-butyl phosphate, and 4 mg/L deoxyribonuclease Evaluation of presence of HLA class I and I antigens Recellularization with patient's ECs and SMCs Vessel implantation After 1st year of implantation, the graft was occluded and a new surgical operation was performed. The second recellularized vascular graft remained patent. No need for immunosuppressive agents	Olausson et al. [195]
HUV	In vivo (large-scale clinical trial)	Stabilized hUV applied in femoropopliteal bypass grafting in 171 patients 6% of the patients died within the 1st year The patency rate was 65% and 50% within the first and fifth year, respectively.	Jarrett and Mahood [214]
HUV	In vitro	HUV denudation either with 0.1% w/v collagenase, hypotonic media, or with gentle gas stream for ECs dehydration Better denudation using stream of gas, according to histological, SEM and biomechanical results	Hoenika et al. [215]
HUA	In vitro and in vivo	Trypsin de-endothelialization of hUVs Development multilayer of PSS/PAH films Implantation as a carotid interposition graft in rabbits. Good patency over 12 weeks. Successful cell infiltration by PECAM$^+$ ECs and α-SMA$^+$ SMCs	Kerdjoudj et al. [206]
HUA	In vitro and in vivo	Decellularized hUAs with CHAPS, SDS, EDTA, and EGM-2 buffers Preservation of ECM structure while no cells were evident. Implantation as acellular abdominal interposition grafts. Thrombus formation, but the vessel lumen did not rupture	Gui et al. [208]
HUA	In vitro and in vivo	Decellularization of hUAs with CHAPS, SDS, and α-MEM with 40% FBS. Good preservation of ECM structure, no cellular or nuclear material, good biomechanical properties. Implantation as common carotid interposition graft. Thrombus formation within 30 days after the implantation. In vivo remodeling of hUAs, elastic fibers production	Mallis et al. [172]

4.5. In Vivo Performance of Decellularized and Cellularized SDVGs

Both decellularized and cellularized SDVGs have been tested in a wide series of experiments, including the evaluation of in vivo performance and biocompatibility [193,216]. It has been shown that decellularized SDVGs lack proper function and are characterized by a high probability of thrombus formation and graft failure [2]. Initially, the exposed collagen, located in the lumen side of the acellular SDVGs, triggers the platelets to aggregate [217]. The first step of this process involves the binding of the soluble form of von Willebrand factor (vWF) with the exposed collagen. Then, and upon vessel exposure to increased shear stress, the platelets are stimulated, leading to large aggregations development through the interaction between platelet glycoprotein (GP) Ib-V-IX receptor and vWF [218]. Furthermore, additional platelet receptors, including GPVI and $\alpha_2\beta_1$, offer more stability to the developing thrombus [219]. Besides, the exposed collagen, fibronectin, and laminin assist in the development of thrombus, through the interaction with platelets' integrins $\alpha_5\beta_1$ and $\alpha_6\beta_1$, respectively [217]. Furthermore, VSMCs contribute significantly to vessel functions. VSMCs is a specific smooth muscle cell subset, located in the tunica media of the vessel wall, responsible for vasoconstriction and vasorelaxation [39]. In these processes, the role of ECs in the regulation of vascular tone is very important. Upon stimulation of ECs, due to high shear stress, the nitric oxide (NO) synthase is activated and increases the NO production, which can cause vasorelaxation. In addition, VSMCs produce high amounts of ECM proteins, including collagen, elastin, and fibronectin, contributing to the regeneration of the injured vessels. An additional important function of VSMCs is the ability to retain the circumferential orientation of the collagen and elastin fibers in the vessel wall [61]. It has been shown that the removal of VSMCs during the decellularization process could alter the alignment of the collagen and elastin fibers. The presence of uncrimped collagen and elastin fibers in decellularized vascular grafts can induce significant alteration to their biomechanical properties, resulting in mismatch compliance between resident and transplanted vessels [212].

On the other hand, cellularized engineered SDVGs are conduits with improved properties, which may result in a more favorable outcome upon implantation. For this purpose, vessel bioreactors such as pulsatile flow or dynamic culture systems, are currently used, which can result in vessel production with uniform coverage of ECs and VSMCs. It has been shown in the literature that recellularized TEVGs are characterized by a lower risk for thrombus formation and graft rejection compared to non-cellularized TEVGs. Zhou et al. [220] reported low neo-intimal formation in recellularized vessels, which were obtained from decellularized canine vessels. In addition, Kaushal et al. [221] and Ma et al. [222] showed that the presence of ECs and VSMCs in the manufactured TEVGs contributed to neo-intimal and neo-medial reconstitution. Row et al. [223] managed to trace the cells used for the recellularization of TEVGs postoperatively. The recellularized TEVGs were implanted as interposition grafts into the coronary artery in female sheep for a time period of three months. In this set of experiments, it was observed that donor cells (used for the recellularization) were gradually substituted by the host cells. Importantly, donor cells represented only 17% and 8% of the total cells after 1 and 8 months postoperatively. Furthermore, no T or B cells were evident in the implanted vessels, indicating that the recellularized vessel favors no immune response [223].

Considering the above data, recellularized TEVGs have greater possibilities to avoid neo-intima formation, thrombus development, and graft failure, and are superior to decellularized vascular grafts. Nevertheless, greater effort regarding the recellularization process must be performed by the research groups worldwide to produce properly functional TEVGs.

5. Manufacturing Methods for the Development of SDVGs

Globally, the increased demand for vascular grafts requires the production of readily available functional transplants, although their large-scale production is a quite challenging task. Currently, there is a wide variety of SDVG manufacturing methods, including tissue-engineering by self-assembly (TESA), electrospinning, and bioprinting [224–226]. Since the first attempts of Weinberg, Bell, and Rosenberg in manufacturing vessel conduits, vascular graft production has been evolved and represents a quite interesting and interdisciplinary research field of the 21st century [33,176]. As has been proposed by Langer and Vaccanti, tissue engineering aims to the production of scaffolds or matrices in order to replace or remove the damaged tissues [227]. In the same way, the development of vascular grafts is characterized by the same principles. A number of different scientific areas must be combined to properly produce a vascular graft, which will replace the damaged one. Nowadays, the production and transplantation of LDVGs have been proven efficient based on the performed clinical trials [1]. On the other hand, the production of fully functional SDVGs is still under the developmental stage, needing further exploration. A few companies have achieved significant progress in the production of readily available SDVGs. Among them, Cryolife, Artegraft, Integra, and Gore are providing ready to use vascular grafts, derived mostly from in-house production (synthetic grafts), animal origin (bovine and porcine vessels), and cadaveric donors (human vessels). However, the clinical utility of vessel transplants requires also the evaluation of alternative methods for the production of vascular grafts. The natural ECM structure and its key mechanical properties are difficult to be reproduced with the aforementioned methods, but significant progress to this direction day by day is made.

5.1. TESA Approach

The TESA approach was developed by the pioneer L'Heureux and aimed at the production of vascular grafts utilizing cell sheets [224]. To achieve this outcome, no supporting vascular scaffolds are required.

The basic concept has relied on the use of cell sheets containing fibroblasts, mesenchymal stromal cells (MSCs), ECs, and VSMCs, which were shaped around a mandrel to produce a tubular formation (Figure 3). Further maturation in the pulsatile bioreactor is required in order to vascular grafts to achieve the prerequisite burst pressure and overall mechanical properties [224,228]. The initial work of L' Heureux et al. [229] involved the cultivation of SMCs and fibroblasts in a standard culture medium contained sodium ascorbate. One month later, the produced sheets were shaped with the use of a tubular mandrel. The same technique was applied for the production of the different layers of the vascular graft. The results of this study were impressive. Specifically, histological analysis revealed the proper localization of the cellular populations, while the burst pressure of the produced vascular conduit was more than 2500 mmHg [229]. Moreover, these vessels were implanted as femoral artery interposition grafts in canine animal models, withstood the blood flow, and met the fundamental requirements of a vascular graft. More experiments also were performed utilizing human cells for the development of vascular grafts and their testing in different animal models. The above results led to the performance of the first clinical trial with TESA-produced TEVGs [229].

Between 2004 and 2007, a multicenter clinical trial was performed in patients who followed hemodialysis [230]. In this study, the vascular grafts were produced from the patient's own cells (fibroblasts and SMCs) utilizing the cell-sheet technique in the same way as previously has been described. The produced grafts were characterized by a mean burst pressure of 3512 mmHg and were used as AVF conduits. The patency rates of the grafts were 78% and 60% after the 1st and 6th months of implantation, respectively. The most observed complications involved the development of aneurism and lumen thrombosis. Despite these drawbacks, this study represents an initial step toward the clinical utility of TESA-produced vascular grafts [230].

5.2. Electrospinning

The electrospinning method comprises the first attempt to mimic the complex structure of natural ECM. This method was introduced in 1930, providing an economical solution for scaffold fabrication [231]. Nowadays, its use has been expanded, thus scaffolds for bone and cartilage regeneration can be manufactured efficiently. Electrospinning has relied on the production of nano- and microfibers derived from a viscoelastic solution, where a high electrostatic force is applied. More specifically, the material that will be electrospun is pumped at a slow rate, ending in a high voltage electrical field [34,232]. This, in turn, leads to charging the polymer material during its exit from the syringe, which results in the production of the Taylor cone. A narrow jet of liquid is generated from the Taylor cone, which is further collected to a specific set up, known as the collector (Figure 3). Finally, the production of a scaffold, characterized by adequate ECM structure and fine-tuning mechanical properties, is produced [2,34]. The formation of the produced fibers is affected by various parameters, which are specific for the material, used each time, including molecular weight, surface tension, density, and viscosity [233]. Except for those, other parameters that can affect the fiber composition mostly include the applied electrostatic field, temperature, humidity, and flow rate of the polymers [233].

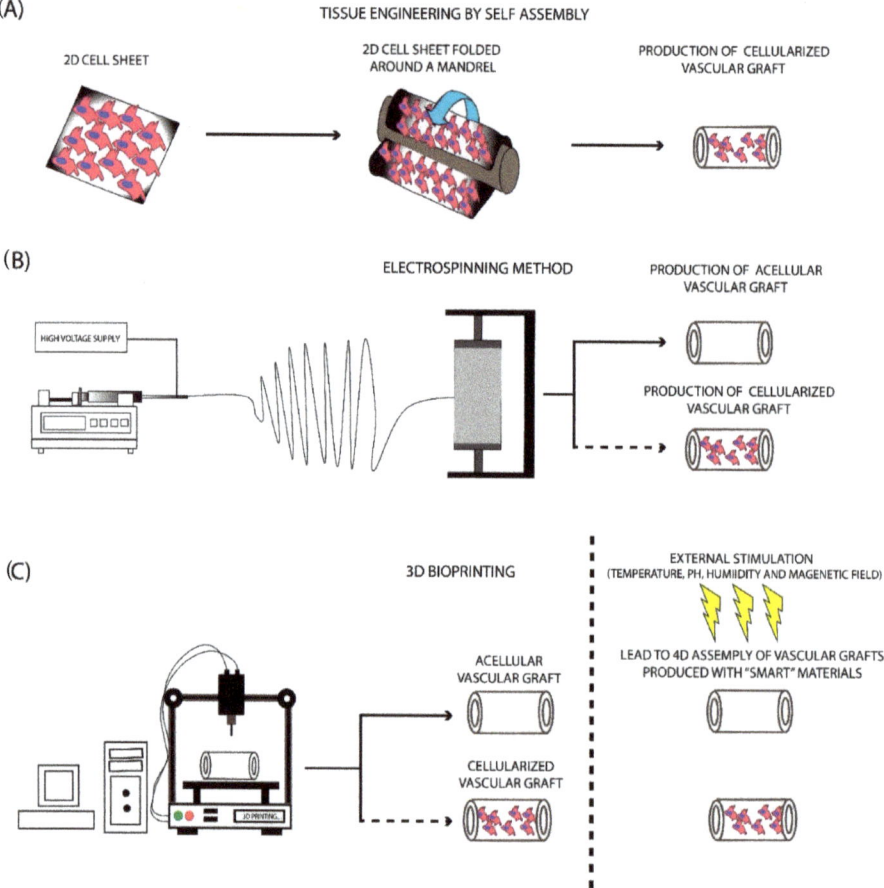

Figure 3. Fabrication methods for the production of SDVGs. (**A**) Production of SDVGs with the originally proposed method of L'Heureux et al. In this method, the production of SDVGs was relied on the self-assembly of cell sheets using a tubular mandrel. (**B**) Production of SDVGs with the electrospinning method. This methodology can produce complicated extracellular matrices (ECMs). In addition, combination with cellular populations can lead to the development of cellularized structures. (**C**) Production of SDVGs with the bioprinting method. Bioprinting offers the potential for the production of either acellular or cellularized complicated structures. Moreover, when used "smart" materials in the production process, the final product can assembly on the desired structure upon external stimulation (e.g., temperature, pH, humidity, and magnetic field).

The polymer materials used in the electrospinning approach could be either degradable or natural derived materials [2,34]. However, important differences between the different materials exist. In the past, degradable materials such as PLA, PGA, PCL, PU/silk fibroin have been used for the production of scaffolds and specifically tubular conduits utilizing the electrospinning approach [2,34]. Vascular grafts have also been fabricated with the electrospinning method. Importantly, the proper combination of PLGA with collagen type I and elastin can improve the mechanical properties of the produced scaffolds, and their use is preferred for the production of electrospun blood vessels [234]. Moreover, it has been shown that the addition of naturally derived materials, such as collagen, gelatin, and fibronectin, may provide more RGD-binding sites, thus improving the cellular functions, like adhesion, growth, and differentiation [235].

In the context of electrospun tubular scaffold application, both acellular and cellularized conduits have been evaluated. Wise et al. [144] developed a tubular scaffold consisted of tropoelastin and PCL with the electrospinning method. The produced scaffold was characterized by similar biomechanical properties as the internal mammary artery (IMA). Further investigation involved the implantation of the acellular conduit in animal models [144]. Furthermore, the biomechanical analysis was performed in electrospun vascular grafts pre- and post-implantation. Specifically, acellular electrospun vascular conduits were implanted as carotid artery interposition grafts in rats for a total period of 1 month. Histological analysis in the explants showed the successful recellularization of the vascular grafts with ECs. Moreover, the explanted electrospun vascular grafts were able to preserve the initial vessel morphology and characterized by similar biomechanical properties as the pre-implanted grafts. In this study, the successful accumulation of tropoelastin in PCL scaffolds was shown for the first time, resulting in the production of vascular grafts, which were characterized by impaired platelet adhesion and increased endothelialization [144]. Additionally, Soletti et al. [236] provided substantial evidence regarding the proper development and production of anti-thrombogenic vascular conduits. Soletti et al. [236] showed that the acellular poly(etherurethane urea) (PEUU) grafts coated with the non-thrombogenic 2-methacryloyloxyethyl phosphorylcholine copolymer showed better patency and mechanical properties compared to uncoated PEUU vascular grafts [236]. Unlike Wise et al. [144] and Soletti et al. [236], Min Ju et al. [237] managed to develop electrospun bilayer tubular scaffolds consisted of PCL and collagen type I. Then, ECs and SMCs obtained from female Dorper Cross Sheep were seeded onto the tubular scaffolds, followed by maturation in the pulsatile flow bioreactor. The seeded vascular grafts were implanted as carotid artery substitutes in the sheep model and remained for 6 months. The electrospun vascular grafts were remained patent and the histological analysis revealed the production of collagen, elastin, and glycosaminoglycans within 6 months of implantation [237]. This study provided valuable data regarding the production and application of the electrospun vascular grafts. Moreover, Du et al. [238] used the electrospinning method to fabricate a 3D vascular microenvironment. In this approach, immobilization of VEGF onto the electrospun tubular scaffold consisted of gradient chitosan and PCL nanofibers was performed. The controlled release of VEGF potentially can enhance the adhesion of ECs and SMCs and further promote their rapid proliferation. In this way, engineered SDVGs with improved anti-thrombogenic properties could be developed, leading to the avoidance of lumen occlusion and thrombus formation, a series of common manifestations which are presented several days after the vessel implantation [238]. Taking into consideration the above data, it was clearly shown that electrospinning could be applied for the efficient production of engineered SDVGs. The produced electrospun SDVGs could be successful in vitro seeded with cellular populations and maintain further their graft patency, mechanical properties, and vessel integrity over a long time period.

5.3. Three Dimensional (3D) Bioprinting

In the last decade, 3D printing technology has gained significant attention and has been utilized with great success in a wide range of applications [239]. Using this technology, complex structures and materials can be produced efficiently, thus can be further used by the scientific society. The evolution of printing technology is 3D bioprinting, which has currently been applied in various tissue engineering approaches [239]. 3D bioprinting can produce complex structures, utilizing non-degradable/degradable and naturally derived polymers [240]. The significant potential of this methodology is the production of ready to use transplantable scaffolds and tissues. Currently, the 3D bioprinting approaches such as inkjet, extrusion, and laser-assisted bioprinting are mostly used for the production of the majority of the scaffolds [240]. A great series of materials are compatible with the bioprinter applications, although the polymer materials are mostly preferred in comparison with the naturally derived materials [240,241]. The bioprinter materials can be distinguished into three categories: (a) fibrous materials, (b) powder materials, and (c) bioinks. The use of the starting material is dependent on the characteristics of the produced scaffold [240,241].

3D bioprinting approaches and the proper combination of the aforementioned materials have been successfully applied in the production of LDVGs and SDVGs. [240,242–244]. In this direction, Freeman et al. [245] presented for the first time a new approach for the development of SDVGs using a custom-made 3D bioprinter. In this study, gelatin and fibrinogen were properly combined, producing a bioink with good rheological and printability properties. The produced vascular graft provided a favorable ECM for cell attachment. However, comprehensive in vitro and in vivo evaluation is further needed to be performed [245]. Jia et al. [246], in their study, used a multilayer coaxial nozzle device to produce vascular grafts. Moreover, human umbilical vein endothelial cells (HUVECs) and MSCs were expanded and encapsulated in a gelatin methacryloyl (GelMA), sodium alginate, and 4-arm poly(ethylene glycol)-tetra-acrylate (PEGTA) based bioink. Using the current bioprinter set-up in combination with the developed bioink resulted in the printing of highly organized vascular structures. No sign of cytotoxicity was reported, and after a time period of 21 days, the cells filled the entire printed vascular grafts. To evaluate better the cell behavior into the vascular wall, immunofluorescence was performed, showing the positive expression of α-SMA and CD31, in MSCs and HUVECs, respectively [246].

5.4. Four-Dimensional (4D) Bioprinting

Next-generation bioprinting demands the use of materials capable of self-transform into a prerequisite shape in order to exert their key functional properties. This state-of-the-art approach is known as 4D bioprinting and has gained increased attention in the last decade by the entire scientific community [247]. 4D bioprinting uses the same materials as conventional 3D printing approaches [240]. The major difference between 3D and 4D bioprinting is that the latter exerts a "smart" behavior of the produced scaffolds [248]. 4D produced scaffolds are superior to the conventionally bioprinted scaffolds. The "smart" behavior corresponds to "materials that can change their physical or chemical properties in a control and functional manner upon exposure to an external stimulus" as has been referred to by Tamay et al. [240]. In this way, 4D printed materials upon exposure to external stimuli such as pH, heat, magnetic field, light, and humidity can adopt effectively different shapes, exhibiting different properties [249]. The above-mentioned factors are playing important role in scaffold's shape-changing properties. There exists a great variety of materials that achieve shape-transformation in response to temperature stimuli. Thermoresponsive materials are the most commonly used in 4D bioprinting applications [250]. These materials can be distinguished into (a) shape memory polymers (SMP) and (b) responsive polymer solutions (RPS). The first category involves polymers consisting of two distinct components, the elastic segment which is characterized by high glass transition temperature (Tg_h), and the switching segment, characterized by intermediate glass transition temperature (Tg_i). When the applied temperature is above the Tg_h, the produced scaffold adopts its permanent shape. On the other hand, when the temperature is between Tg_i and Tg_h, the switching segment becomes soft, while the elastic segment resists any shape-changing [251]. Additionally, if the material is cooled below the Tg_h, then the elastic segment cannot return to its initial shape and the produced scaffolds acquire its final definitive form. SMPs include mostly the poly(ε-caprolactone) dimethacrylate (PCLDMA), polycaprolactone triol (Ptriol), and poly(ether urethane) (PEU). These materials have been used mostly in applications such as bone and cartilage engineering. RPS is characterized by a critical solution temperature, where if the applied temperature is above the aforementioned temperature (critical solution temperature), the polymer chains are contracting and the overall solution is adopting a solid form [247].

Both hydrophobic and hydrophilic interactions are existing between the polymer chains. In addition, a change in temperature may affect the behavior and the interaction of the above polymer chains. This, in turn, leads to shrinkage or expansion, which is a characteristic of each polymer material. In this direction, a material with a critical solution temperature above 25°C, when implanted to a mammalian organism, would expand, acquiring its definitive form. Poly(N-isopropylacrylamide), poly(ethylene glycol), collagen, gelatin, and methylcellulose are some of the most used RPS [249].

Besides the temperature stimuli, materials that can respond to pH changes also can be widely applied in the clinical setting [247]. The initial structure of these materials is consisting of acidic or basic groups, which are the main players in proton exchange upon pH changes [252]. In this way, polymers consisting of acidic groups, when exposed to pH > 7, act as anionic compounds, while polymers with a basic group, exposed to pH < 7, act as cationic compounds. Therefore, these materials upon pH stimuli can acquire different structural and functional properties, including change in solubility, degradability, swelling, etc. [248]. Like thermoresponsive polymers, pH-responsive polymers also can be utilized in a wide range of applications. Indeed, different human body compartments are characterized by different pH in order to serve properly their initial function, including the gastrointestinal tract, stomach, small intestine, and different regions of the vascular system including the kidney vascular network. Additionally, many solid tumors induce pH changes upon their growth. In this way, pH-responsive polymers can act as DDS, delivering tumor-specific therapy, such as signaling and cell proliferation inhibitors or monoclonal antibodies [253]. Examples of the most commonly used materials in this category are poly(acrylic acid), poly(aspartic acid), poly(L-glutamic acid), and poly(histidine), which can be combined effectively with naturally derived materials such as collagen, gelatin, and chitosan [252].

Besides the aforementioned, other categories of responsive materials have also been manufactured. These categories mostly include the photoresponsive, magneto-responsive, and humidity-responsive materials. However, their potential use is limited and, therefore, further evaluation of their properties is clearly needed. Briefly, photoresponsive materials can change their structural and functional properties, including wettability, solubility, degradability upon photo-stimulation [240]. Considering this, polymer materials with photosensitive groups can be manufactured, where the produced scaffolds can swell or shrink when specific photo-stimulation is applied. The combination of magnetic particles with polymer materials results in the development of magneto-responsive materials. The most commonly used magnetic particles are iron (Fe), nickel (Ni), cobalt (Co), and their oxides [249] Currently, magneto-responsive materials have been used as targeted therapeutic vehicles, carrying anti-tumor drugs. On the other hand, significant adverse reactions may be induced by their use in living organisms [254]. It has been shown that magnetic particles with a size less than 50 nm are transportable through the biological matrix, which can further cause inflammation and cell death due to high reactive oxygen species (ROS) production, DNA damage, and cytochrome C release. In this category, materials such as Fe_3O_4/PCL, Fe_3O_4/poly (ethylene glycol diacrylate), PCL/iron doped hydroxyapatite (PCL/FeHA) are currently evaluated for their potent use in living systems [254]. Lastly, humidity responsive materials also have been proposed for their use in 4D bioprinting and the production of tissue-engineered scaffolds. Interestingly the change in humidity could result in shape-change modification, which can act as a driving force for movement. These materials have not received great attention from the scientific community due to their limited use. Humidity responsive materials include poly(ethylene glycol) diacrylate, cellulose, polyurethane, and their combinations [255].

The 4D bioprinting comprises an important evolution in the fabrication of tissue-engineered scaffolds. Vascular grafts can be developed with this next-generation approach. In this way, we can imagine the development of a 4D bioprinted vascular graft (with a large or small diameter), which can acquire its specific shape inside the living organism upon temperature stimulation. Moreover, changes in pH of the vascular network may stimulate the implanted vascular graft in a way either to acquire a different shape or to substantially release key therapeutic agents in order to reduce or even to reverse the occurred situation. In the future, "smart" telebiometrics vascular grafts will be plausible to be employed, which can detect the changes of human body conditions, like temperature, pH, osmolarity, and will be able to notify or even to reverse a health issue. Currently, the utilization of "smart" materials and the manufacturing of those scaffolds is under the developmental stage [247]. Therefore, no significant number of publications is currently existing, with the only exceptions of reviews and opinion articles in this field. In this way, the development of "smart" materials that can be used in vascular engineering is quite important, but further exploration of this research field is needed.

6. Concluding Remarks

Globally, there is an increasing demand for SDVGs, as they are employed primarily in cardiovascular reconstruction surgeries. Indeed, more than 400,000 bypass surgeries are performed each year [12–15]. Parameters such as the modern way of life, increased working hours, overall stress, lack of physical exercise, and smoking comprise important risk factors for CVD development [18,20]. From an economical point of view, CVD is also a serious burden for all countries; therefore, novel and better treatment options must be utilized [21]. In this direction, the production of SDVGs and their efficient application in patients suffering from disorders that are belonging to CVD could be an important alternative strategy. One of the applied therapeutic approaches that are currently followed is the replacement of damaged vessels with autologous vascular grafts, such as the SV, mammary artery, and others [208]. However, CVD can affect the entire circulatory system, therefore, less than 60% of the patients have suitable vessels. Moreover, when second vascular reconstruction is needed to be performed in the same patient, this percentage is lower than 15% [31]. Blood vessel compatibility is another important parameter that should have in mind. Compliance mismatch between native and implanted graft (mostly at the anastomosis site) could induce unfavorable results, including calcification initiation, intima hyperplasia, lumen occlusion, platelets aggregation, and thrombus formation [32]. To avoid the above manifestations and in order to the availability of the vascular grafts to be increased, alternative strategies must be explored. Currently, the fabrication of LDVGs is efficient, using the latest TE approaches; therefore, the utilization of these methods could be applied in SDVGs production [2]. Although the significant drawbacks which engineered SDVGs may present, the interest of the scientific society is increasing day by day, exploiting better strategies to improve further the development of those grafts. Nowadays, the production of the SDVGs relies on the use of synthetic (non-degradable/degradable), naturally derived materials, and decellularized ECM. These materials can be combined with state-of-the-art manufacturing approaches (TESA, electrospinning, bioprinting) to produce vascular grafts with improved properties [2,245]. In most of these approaches, cell seeding and maturation in bioreactors (mostly pulsatile flow bioreactors) are needed in order to produced vascular grafts to effectively cellularized and acquire the proper biomechanical properties. Additionally, the decellularization of tissues and organs is a very promising approach, especially for the development of SDVGs. Indeed, decellularization can efficiently be applied in vessels such as the umbilical arteries or vessels derived from cadaveric donors to produce properly defined SDVGs.

In vascular engineering, different cellular populations have been proposed such as ECs, VSMCs, and stem cells, derived mostly from the recipient, avoiding in this way any unfavorable immune response and possibly graft failure and rejection [34]. However, a great number of cellular populations are needed for tissue engineering approaches. Terminally differentiated cells such as ECs and VSMCs can be isolated from a vessel biopsy, although to reach cell numbers >10×10^7 requires extended in vitro manipulation and cultivation. On the other hand, the use of stem cells such as Mesenchymal Stromal Cells (MSCs) may be a more feasible approach. MSCs initially were isolated from bone marrow aspirates, while currently other sources including the adipose tissue and stromal vascular fraction can be used [256,257]. MSCs is a heterogenic multipotent stem cell population derived from mesoderm, and capable to differentiate effectively to "chondrocytes", "adipocytes", and "osteocytes" [258]. Immunophenotypically, these cells express (>95%) CD73, CD90, and CD105, while lacking the expression (<3%) of CD34, CD45, and HLA-DR, as has been indicated by MSCs committee of the International Society of Cell and Gene Therapy (ISCT) [259]. MSCs can be easily in vitro handled, while their stemness (specific gene expression and protein production) can be retained for an increased number of passages (>P8). Another candidate stem cell population for vascular engineering may be the induced pluripotent stem cells (iPSCs). In 2006, for the first time, Shinya Yamanaka managed to gain the pluripotent state of terminally differentiated cells by introducing a set of specific genes, including OCT4, SOX3, KLF4, and C-MYC [260]. Currently, different strategies have been developed for the production of iPSCs, even avoiding the use of *C-MYC*, a known oncogene. The efficient differentiation of iPSCs into various cell populations such as neural cells, cardiomyocytes, hepatic cells, ECs, VSMCs, etc. has been demonstrated in literature [261,262]. However, this technology has not yet received FDA approval for human clinical use, and therefore their applicability is limited even in vascular engineering [263,264].

The cellularization of TEVGs comprises a crucial step in the manufacturing process. Indeed, it has been shown that cell-seeded vascular grafts are characterized by better integration properties in the recipient's body [2]. In this way, properly cellularized vascular grafts can avoid the interaction with M1 macrophages, favoring in this way the attraction of M2 macrophages. M2 macrophages have been related to the tissue remodeling process, avoiding the activation of T and B cells [265]. Moreover, several research groups have observed the development of vasa vasorum, the responsible vessels for nutrient supplementation, into the transplanted vascular grafts, indicating its further proper adaptation by the studied living system [172,266].

The proper manufacturing of SDVGs is an important aspect, and for this purpose, specific evaluation tests must be performed before their final application. These tests include (a) histological analysis, (b) biochemical and DNA quantification, (c) cytotoxicity assay, (d) platelet adhesion assays, (e) biomechanical analysis, and (f) implantation in animal models in order to assess effectively functionality of the vascular grafts. The above processes represent the first line of evaluation tests that should be performed to assess the biocompatibility of the manufactured SDVGs. Furthermore, more tests need to be performed to properly define the produced TEVGs. Especially for the SDVGs, the performance of cytotoxicity and the platelet adhesion assays is of major importance. In contrast to LDVGs, manufactured SDVGs are characterized by an increased probability of platelet aggregation and thrombus formation. Moreover, ECs should be properly seeded in SDVGs to produce a functional endothelium; therefore, the establishment of a non-toxic vascular graft is highly recommended.

Taking into consideration the above information of this review, we can conclude that the production of SDVGs is requiring further improvement, which is performed by several research groups worldwide. Currently, the use of synthetic and decellularized vascular grafts has gained a significant advantage over other methods. Highly organized ECMs cannot be in detail reproduced with the bioprinting approaches. Indeed, additive manufacturing techniques such as 3D and 4D bioprinting are characterized by a few limitations. The inability of reproducing the highly organized structure of SDVGs may comprise the most significant drawback of the current approaches. SDVGs are characterized by a complex structure, where collagen, elastin, fibronectin, and other key ECM proteins have specific relation and orientation in the vascular wall, ensuring in this way the proper recellularization. Cellularization of the bioprinted vessel constructs may be related to improved biocompatibility and biomechanical properties. In order to produce highly organized constructs, crosslinking of the biomaterials, used in bioprinting approaches, is preferred. However, the use of fixative agents such as glutaraldehyde, can result in increased cytotoxicity and altered biomechanical properties to the produced vascular scaffolds [103,205]. Moreover, when naturally derived bioinks are used, crosslinking may hamper the in vivo remodeling process of the vascular graft, leading to unfavorable outcomes. Moreover, the manufacturing of vessel constructs with high resolution demands high-cost printing devices and experienced personnel. Besides these drawbacks, in the future, the quality of bioprinters and printed constructs will be improved, leading to a new era in SDVGs development. Besides the above limitations, the introduction of 3D and 4D printing approaches may represent a new era regarding vascular scaffold production [240,247].

In conclusion, SDVGs now can be robustly produced and can be used in personalized medicine. Each production step must be specifically evaluated and the overall process must be performed in compliance with Good Manufacturing Practices (GMPs) conditions in order to produce readily available safe and fully functional grafts for patients suffering from CVD.

Author Contributions: Conceptualization, writing—original draft preparation, visualization, writing—review and editing, P.M.; supervision, project administration, C.S.-G. and A.K.; conceptualization, writing—review and editing, supervision, project administration, E.M. All authors have read and agreed to the published version of the manuscript.

Funding: This research received no external funding.

Conflicts of Interest: The authors declare no conflict of interest.

References

1. Matsuzaki, Y.; John, K.; Shoji, T.; Shinoka, T. The Evolution of Tissue Engineered Vascular Graft Technologies: From Preclinical Trials to Advancing Patient Care. *Appl. Sci.* **2019**, *9*, 1274. [CrossRef] [PubMed]
2. Pashneh-Tala, S.; MacNeil, S.; Claeyssens, F. The Tissue-Engineered Vascular Graft-Past, Present, and Future. *Tissue Eng. Part B Rev.* **2016**, *22*, 68–100. [CrossRef]
3. Ong, C.S.; Zhou, X.; Huang, C.Y.; Fukunishi, T.; Zhang, H.; Hibino, N. Tissue engineered vascular grafts: Current state of the field. *Expert Rev. Med. Devices* **2017**, *14*, 383–392. [CrossRef]
4. Xue, L.; Greisler, H.P. Biomaterials in the development and future of vascular grafts. *J. Vasc. Surg.* **2003**, *37*, 472–480. [CrossRef] [PubMed]
5. Clupac, J.; Filova, E.; Bacakova, L. Blood vessel replacement: 50 years of development and tissue engineering paradigms in vascular surgery. *Physiol. Res.* **2009**, *58*, s119–s139.
6. Brewster, D.C. Current controversies in the management of aortoiliac occlusive disease. *J. Vasc. Surg.* **1997**, *25*, 365–379. [CrossRef]
7. Hadinata, I.E.; Hayward, P.A.; Hare, D.L.; Matalanis, G.S.; Seevanayagam, S.; Rosalion, A.; Buxton, B.F. Choice of conduit for the right coronary system: 8-year analysis of Radial Artery Patency and Clinical Outcomes trial. *Ann. Thorac. Surg.* **2009**, *88*, 1404–1409. [CrossRef]
8. Zoghbi, W.A.; Duncan, T.; Antman, E.; Barbosa, M.; Champagne, B.; Chen, D.; Gamra, H.; Harold, J.G.; Josephson, S.; Komajda, M.; et al. Sustainable development goals and the future of cardiovascular health: A statement from the Global Cardiovascular Disease Taskforce. *Glob. Heart* **2014**, *9*, 273–274. [CrossRef]
9. Matters, C.D.; Loncar, D. Projections of Global Mortality and Burden of Disease from 2002 to 2030. *PLoS Med.* **2006**, *3*, e442. [CrossRef]
10. Abdulhannan, P.; Russell, D.A.; Homer-Vanniasinkam, S. Peripheral arterial disease: A literature review. *Br. Med. Bull.* **2012**, *104*, 21–39. [CrossRef]
11. European Cardiovascular Disease Statistics. Available online: http://www.ehnheart.org/cvd-statistics.html (accessed on 25 October 2020).
12. Movsisyan, N.K.; Vinciguerra, M.; Medina-Inojosa, J.R.; Lopez-Jimenez, F. Cardiovascular Diseases in Central and Eastern Europe: A Call for More Surveillance and Evidence-Based Health Promotion. *Ann. Glob. Health* **2020**, *86*, 21. [CrossRef] [PubMed]
13. World Health Organization. Available online: https://www.euro.who.int/en/health-topics/noncommunicable-diseases/cardiovascular-diseases (accessed on 25 October 2020).
14. Mensah, G.A.; Brown, D.W. An overview of cardiovascular disease burden in the United States. *Health Aff.* **2007**, *26*, 38–48. [CrossRef] [PubMed]
15. Heart and Stroke Statistics. Available online: https://www.heart.org/en/about-us/heart-and-stroke-association-statistics (accessed on 25 October 2020).
16. Thom, T.; Haase, N.; Rosamond, W.; Howard, V.J.; Rumsfeld, J.; Manolio, T.; Zheng, Z.J.; Flegal, K.; O'Donnell, C.; Kittner, S.; et al. American Heart Association Statistics, C.; Stroke Statistics, S. Heart disease and stroke statistics—2006 update: A report from the American Heart Association Statistics Committee and Stroke Statistics Subcommittee. *Circulation* **2006**, *113*, e85–e151. [PubMed]

17. Noly, P.E.; Ben Ali, W.; Lamarche, Y.; Carrier, M. Status, Indications, and Use of Cardiac Replacement Therapy in the Era of Multimodal Mechanical Approaches to Circulatory Support: A Scoping Review. *Can. J. Cardiol.* **2020**, *36*, 261–269. [CrossRef]
18. Ditano-Vazquez, P.; Torres-Pena, J.D.; Galeano-Valle, F.; Perez-Caballero, A.I.; Demelo-Rodriguez, P.; Lopez-Miranda, J.; Katsiki, N.; Delgado-Lista, J.; Alvarez-Sala-Walther, L.A. The Fluid Aspect of the Mediterranean Diet in the Prevention and Management of Cardiovascular Disease and Diabetes: The Role of Polyphenol Content in Moderate Consumption of Wine and Olive Oil. *Nutrients* **2019**, *11*, 2833. [CrossRef]
19. World Health Organization. Cardiovascular Diseases. Available online: https://www.who.int/news-room/fact-sheets/detail/cardiovascular-diseases-(cvds) (accessed on 25 October 2020).
20. Maniadakis, N.; Kourlaba, G.; Fragoulakis, V. Self-reported prevalence of atherothrombosis in a general population sample of adults in Greece; A telephone survey. *BMC Cardiovasc. Disord.* **2011**, *11*, 16. [CrossRef]
21. Maniadakis, N.; Kourlaba, G.; Angeli, A.; Kyriopoulos, J. The economic burden if atherothrombosis in Greece: Results from the THESIS study. *Eur. J. Health Econ.* **2013**, *14*, 655–665. [CrossRef]
22. Sanchez, P.F.; Brey, E.M.; Briceno, J.C. Endothelialization mechanisms in vascular grafts. *J. Tissue Eng. Regen. Med.* **2018**, *12*, 2164–2178. [CrossRef]
23. Cheng, D.; Allen, K.; Cohn, W.; Connolly, M.; Edgerton, J.; Falk, V.; Martin, J.; Ohtsuka, T.; Vitali, R. Endoscopic vascular harvest in coronary artery bypass grafting surgery: A meta-analysis of randomized trials and controlled trials. *Innovations* **2005**, *1*, 61–74. [CrossRef]
24. Björk, V.O.; Ekeström, S.; Henze, A.; Ivert, T.; Landou, C. Early and Late Patency of Aortocoronary Vein Grafts. *Scand. J. Thorac. Cardiovasc. Surg.* **1981**, *15*, 11–21. [CrossRef]
25. Widimsky, P.; Straka, Z.; Stros, P.; Jirasek, K.; Dvorak, J.; Votava, J.; Lisa, L.; Budesinsky, T.; Kolesar, M.; Vanek, T.; et al. One-Year Coronary Bypass Graft Patency. *Circulation* **2004**, *110*, 3418–3423. [CrossRef] [PubMed]
26. Fitzgibbon, G.M.; Kafka, H.P.; Leach, A.J.; Keon, W.J.; Hooper, G.D.; Burton, J.R. Coronary bypass graft fate and patient outcome: Angiographic follow-up of 5065 grafts related to survival and reoperation in 1,388 patients during 25 years. *J. Am. Coll. Cardiol.* **1996**, *28*, 616–626. [CrossRef]
27. Gaudino, M.; Benedetto, U.; Fremes, S.; Biondi-Zoccai, G.; Sedrakyan, A.; Puskas, J.D.; Angelini, G.D.; Buxton, B.; Frati, G.; Hare, D.L.; et al. Radial-Artery or Saphenous-Vein Grafts in Coronary-Artery Bypass Surgery. *N. Engl. J. Med.* **2018**, *378*, 2069–2077. [CrossRef] [PubMed]
28. Menzoian, J.O.; Koshar, A.L.; Rodrigues, N. Alexis Carrel, Rene Leriche, Jean Kunlin, and the history of bypass surgery. *J. Vasc. Surg.* **2011**, *54*, 571–574. [CrossRef]
29. Shah, P.J.; Bui, K.; Blackmore, S.; Gordon, I.; Hare, D.L.; Fuller, J.; Seevanayagam, S.; Buxton, B.F. Has the in situ right internal thoracic artery been overlooked? An angiographic study of the radial artery, internal thoracic arteries and saphenous vein graft patencies in symptomatic patients. *Eur. J. Cardio-Thorac. Surg.* **2005**, *27*, 870–875. [CrossRef]
30. Chard, R.B.; Johnson, D.C.; Nunn, G.R.; Cartmill, T.B. Aorta-coronary bypass grafting with polytetrafluoroethylene conduits. Early and late outcome in eight patients. *J. Thorac. Cardiovasc. Surg.* **1987**, *94*, 132–134. [CrossRef]
31. Popov, G.; Vavilov, V.; Popryaduhin, P. Is it Possible to Create Readily Available Tissue-Engineered Vascular Grafts Without Using Cells? *Eur. J. Vasc. Endovasc. Surg.* **2019**, *58*, e190–e191. [CrossRef]
32. Patterson, J.; Gilliland, T.; Maxfield, M.; Church, S.; Naito, Y.; Shinoka, T.; Breuer, C.K. Tissue-engineered vascular grafts for use in the treatment of congenital heart disease: From the bench to the clinic and back again. *Reg. Med.* **2012**, *7*, 409–419. [CrossRef]
33. Weinberg, C.B.; Bell, E. A blood vessel model constructed from collagen and cultured vascular cells. *Science* **1986**, *231*, 397–400. [CrossRef]
34. Carrabba, M.; Madeddu, P. Current Strategies for the Manufacture of Small Size Tissue Engineering Vascular Grafts. *Front. Bioeng. Biotechnol.* **2018**, *6*, 41. [CrossRef]
35. Mirensky, T.L.; Hibino, N.; Sawh-Martinez, R.F.; Yi, T.; Villalona, G.; Shinoka, T.; Breuer, C.K. Tissue-engineered vascular grafts: Does cell seeding matter? *J. Pediatric Surg.* **2010**, *45*, 1299–1305. [CrossRef] [PubMed]
36. Lin, C.H.; Hsia, K.; Ma, H.; Lee, H.; Lu, J.H. In Vivo Performance of Decellularized Vascular Grafts: A Review Article. *Int. J. Mol. Sci.* **2018**, *19*, 2101. [CrossRef] [PubMed]
37. Michiels, C. Endothelial cell functions. *J. Cell. Physiol.* **2003**, *196*, 430–443. [CrossRef] [PubMed]

38. Feletou, M. The Endothelium: Part 1: Multiple Functions of the Endothelial Cells—Focus on Endothelium-Derived Vasoactive Mediators. *Morgan Claypool Life Sci.* **2011**, *3*, 1–306.
39. Mallis, P.; Papapanagiotou, A.; Katsimpoulas, M.; Kostakis, A.; Siasos, G.; Kassi, E.; Stavropoulos-Giokas, C.; Michalopoulos, E. Efficient differentiation of vascular smooth muscle cells from Wharton's Jelly mesenchymal stromal cells using human platelet lysate: A potential cell source for small blood vessel engineering. *World J. Stem Cells* **2020**, *12*, 203–221. [CrossRef] [PubMed]
40. Zhang, W.J.; Liu, W.; Cui, L.; Cao, Y. Tissue engineering of blood vessel. *J. Cell. Mol. Med.* **2007**, *11*, 945–957. [CrossRef] [PubMed]
41. Knight, D.K.; Gillies, E.R.; Mequanint, K. Vascular Grafting Strategies in Coronary Intervention. *Front. Mater.* **2014**, *1*, 4. [CrossRef]
42. Hashi, C.K.; Derugin, N.; Janairo, R.R.; Lee, R.; Schultz, D.; Lotz, J.; Li, S. Antithrombogenic modification of small-diameter microfibrous vascular grafts. *Arterioscler. Thromb. Vasc. Biol.* **2010**, *30*, 1621–1627. [CrossRef]
43. Radke, D.; Jia, W.; Sharma, D.; Fena, K.; Wang, G.; Goldman, J.; Zhao, F. Tissue Engineering at the Blood-Contacting Surface: A Review of Challenges and Strategies in Vascular Graft Development. *Adv. Healthc. Mater.* **2018**, *7*, e1701461. [CrossRef]
44. Yuan, H.; Chen, C.; Liu, Y.; Lu, T.; Wu, Z. Strategies in cell-free tissue-engineered vascular grafts. *J. Biomed. Mater. Res. Part A* **2020**, *108*, 426–445. [CrossRef]
45. Ku, D.N.; Han, H.-C. Assessment of Function in Tissue-Engineered Vascular Grafts. In *Functional Tissue Engineering*; Guilak, F., Butler, D.L., Goldstein, S.A., Mooney, D.J., Eds.; Springer: New York, NY, USA, 2003; pp. 258–267.
46. Atlan, M.; Simon-Yarza, T.; Ino, J.M.; Hunsinger, V.; Corte, L.; Ou, P.; Aid-Launais, R.; Chaouat, M.; Letourneur, D. Design, characterization and in vivo performance of synthetic 2 mm-diameter vessel grafts made of PVA-gelatin blends. *Sci. Rep.* **2018**, *8*, 7417. [CrossRef]
47. Ravi, S.; Qu, Z.; Chaikof, E.L. Polymeric materials for tissue engineering of arterial substitutes. *Vascular* **2009**, *17* (Suppl. 1), S45–S54. [CrossRef]
48. Ravi, S.; Chaikof, E.L. Biomaterials for vascular tissue engineering. *Regen. Med.* **2010**, *5*, 107–120. [CrossRef] [PubMed]
49. Campbell, C.D.; Brooks, D.H.; Webster, M.W.; Bahnson, H.T. The use of expanded microporous polytetrafluoroethylene for limb salvage: A preliminary report. *Surgery* **1976**, *79*, 485–491. [PubMed]
50. McAuley, C.E.; Steed, D.L.; Webster, M.W. Seven-year follow-up of expanded polytetrafluoroethylene (PTFE) femoropopliteal bypass grafts. *Ann. Surg.* **1984**, *199*, 57–60. [CrossRef] [PubMed]
51. Goldman, M.; McCollum, C.N.; Hawker, R.J.; Drolc, Z.; Slaney, G. Dacron arterial grafts: The influence of porosity, velour, and maturity on thrombogenicity. *Surgery* **1982**, *92*, 947–952. [PubMed]
52. Lodi, M.; Cavallini, G.; Susa, A.; Lanfredi, M. Biomaterials and immune system: Cellular reactivity towards PTFE and Dacron vascular substitutes pointed out by the leukocyte adherence inhibition (LAI) test. *Int. Angiol.* **1988**, *7*, 344–348.
53. Mitchell, R.N. Graft vascular disease: Immune response meets the vessel wall. *Annu. Rev. Pathol.* **2009**, *4*, 19–47. [CrossRef] [PubMed]
54. Antonova, L.V.; Silnikov, V.N.; Sevostyanova, V.V.; Yuzhalin, A.E.; Koroleva, L.S.; Velikanova, E.A.; Mironov, A.V.; Godovikova, T.S.; Kutikhin, A.G.; Glushkova, T.V.; et al. Biocompatibility of Small-Diameter Vascular Grafts in Different Modes of RGD Modification. *Polymers* **2019**, *11*, 174. [CrossRef]
55. Li, C.; Hill, A.; Imran, M. In vitro and in vivo studies of ePTFE vascular grafts treated with P15 peptide. *J. Biomater. Sci. Polym. Ed.* **2005**, *16*, 875–891. [CrossRef]
56. Heidenhain, C.; Veeravoorn, A.; Vachkov, B.; Weichert, W.; Schmidmaier, G.; Wildemann, B.; Neuhaus, P.; Heise, M. Fibroblast and vascular endothelial growth factor coating of decellularized vascular grafts stimulates undesired giant cells and graft encapsulation in a rat model. *Artif. Organs* **2011**, *35*, E1–E10. [CrossRef] [PubMed]
57. Lahtinen, M.; Blomberg, P.; Baliulis, G.; Carlsson, F.; Khamis, H.; Zemgulis, V. In vivo h-VEGF165 gene transfer improves early endothelialisation and patency in synthetic vascular grafts. *Eur. J. Cardio-Thorac. Surg.* **2007**, *31*, 383–390. [CrossRef] [PubMed]
58. McClure, M.J.; Wolfe, P.S.; Rodriguez, I.A.; Bowlin, G.L. Bioengineered vascular grafts: Improving vascular tissue engineering through scaffold design. *J. Drug Deliv. Sci. Technol.* **2011**, *21*, 211–227. [CrossRef]

59. Randone, B.; Cavallaro, G.; Polistena, A.; Cucina, A.; Coluccia, P.; Graziano, P.; Cavallaro, A. Dual role of VEGF in pretreated experimental ePTFE arterial grafts. *J. Surg. Res.* **2005**, *127*, 70–79. [CrossRef]
60. Suzuki, Y.; Montagne, K.; Nishihara, A.; Watabe, T.; Miyazono, K. BMPs promote proliferation and migration of endothelial cells via stimulation of VEGF-A/VEGFR2 and angiopoietin-1/Tie2 signalling. *J. Biochem.* **2008**, *143*, 199–206. [CrossRef]
61. Milliat, F.; Francois, A.; Isoir, M.; Deutsch, E.; Tamarat, R.; Tarlet, G.; Atfi, A.; Validire, P.; Bourhis, J.; Sabourin, J.C.; et al. Influence of endothelial cells on vascular smooth muscle cells phenotype after irradiation: Implication in radiation-induced vascular damages. *Am. J. Pathol.* **2006**, *169*, 1484–1495. [CrossRef]
62. Kakisis, J.D.; Liapis, C.D.; Breuer, C.; Sumpio, B.E. Artificial blood vessel: The Holy Grail of peripheral vascular surgery. *J. Vasc. Surg.* **2005**, *41*, 349–354. [CrossRef]
63. Hamilos, M.; Petousis, S.; Parthenakis, F. Interaction between platelets and endothelium: From pathophysiology to new therapeutic options. *Cardiovasc. Diagn. Ther.* **2018**, *8*, 568–580. [CrossRef]
64. Hoshi, R.A.; Van Lith, R.; Jen, M.C.; Allen, J.B.; Lapidos, K.A.; Ameer, G. The blood and vascular cell compatibility of heparin-modified ePTFE vascular grafts. *Biomaterials* **2013**, *34*, 30–41. [CrossRef]
65. Sugawara, Y.; Miyata, T.; Sato, O.; Kimura, H.; Namba, T.; Makuuchi, M. Rapid postincubation endothelial retention by Dacron grafts. *J. Surg. Res.* **1997**, *67*, 132–136. [CrossRef]
66. Phaneuf, M.D.; Dempsey, D.J.; Bide, M.J.; Quist, W.C.; LoGerfo, F.W. Coating of Dacron vascular grafts with an ionic polyurethane: A novel sealant with protein binding properties. *Biomterilas* **2001**, *22*, 463–469. [CrossRef]
67. Hytonen, J.P.; Leppanen, O.; Taavitsainen, J.; Korpisalo, P.; Laidinen, S.; Alitalo, K.; Wadstrom, J.; Rissanen, T.T.; Yla-Herttuala, S. Improved endothelialization of small-diameter ePTFE vascular grafts through growth factor therapy. *Vasc. Biol.* **2019**, *1*, 1–9. [CrossRef] [PubMed]
68. Mall, J.W.; Philipp, A.W.; Rademacher, A.; Paulitschke, M.; Buttemeyer, R. Re-endothelialization of punctured ePTFE graft: An in vitro study under pulsed perfusion conditions. *Nephrol. Dial. Transplant.* **2004**, *19*, 61–67. [CrossRef] [PubMed]
69. Sipehia, R.; Liszkowski, M.; Lu, A. In vivo evaluation of ammonia plasma modified ePTFE grafts for small diameter blood vessels replacement. A preliminary report. *J. Cardiovasc. Surg.* **2001**, *42*, 537–542.
70. Zhang, Z.; Wang, Z.; Liu, S.; Kodama, M. Pore size, tissue ingrowth, and endothelialization of small-diameter microporous polyurethane vascular prostheses. *Biomaterials* **2004**, *25*, 177–187. [CrossRef]
71. Chandy, T.; Das, G.S.; Wilson, R.F.; Rao, G.H. Use of plasma glow for surface-engineering biomolecules to enhance bloodcompatibility of Dacron and PTFE vascular prosthesis. *Biomaterials* **2000**, *21*, 699–712. [CrossRef]
72. Hirko, M.K.; Schmidt, S.P.; Hunter, T.J.; Evancho, M.M.; Sharp, W.V.; Donovan, D.L. Endothelial cell seeding improves 4 mm PTFE vascular graft performance in antiplatelet medicated dogs. *Artery* **1987**, *14*, 137–153.
73. Lewitus, D.Y.; Rios, F.; Rojas, R.; Kohn, J. Molecular design and evaluation of biodegradable polymers using a statistical approach. *J. Mater. Sci. Mater. Med.* **2013**, *24*, 2529–2535. [CrossRef]
74. Kulkarni, R.K.; Pani, K.C.; Neuman, C.; Leonard, F. Polylactic acid for surgical implants. *Arch. Surg.* **1966**, *93*, 839–843. [CrossRef]
75. Tallawi, M.; Rosellini, E.; Barbani, N.; Cascone, M.G.; Rai, R.; Saint-Pierre, G.; Boccaccini, A.R. Strategies for the chemical and biological functionalization of scaffolds for cardiac tissue engineering: A review. *J. R. Soc. Interface* **2015**, *12*, 20150254. [CrossRef]
76. He, W.; Yong, T.; Teo, W.E.; Ma, Z.; Ramakrishna, S. Fabrication and endothelialization of collagen-blended biodegradable polymer nanofibers: Potential vascular graft for blood vessel tissue engineering. *Tissue Eng.* **2005**, *11*, 1574–1588. [CrossRef] [PubMed]
77. Wang, S.; Zhang, Y.; Yin, G.; Wang, H.; Dong, Z. Electrospun polylactide/silk fibroin-gelatin composite tubular scaffolds for small-diameter tissue engineering blood vessels. *J. Appl. Polym. Sci.* **2009**, *113*, 2675–2682. [CrossRef]
78. Quint, C.; Arief, M.; Muto, A.; Dardik, A.; Niklason, L.E. Allogeneic human tissue-engineered blood vessel. *J. Vasc. Surg.* **2012**, *55*, 790–798. [CrossRef] [PubMed]
79. Lawson, J.H.; Glickman, M.H.; Ilzecki, M.; Jakimowicz, T.; Jaroszynski, A.; Peden, E.K.; Pilgrim, A.J.; Prichard, H.L.; Guziewicz, M.; Przywara, S.; et al. Bioengineered human acellular vessels for dialysis access in patients with end-stage renal disease: Two phase 2 single-arm trials. *Lancet* **2016**, *387*, 2026–2034. [CrossRef]

80. Antonova, L.V.; Mironov, A.V.; Yuzhalin, A.E.; Krivkina, E.O.; Shabaev, A.R.; Rezvova, M.A.; Tkachenko, V.O.; Khanova, M.Y.; Sergeeva, T.Y.; Krutitskiy, S.S.; et al. A Brief Report on an Implantation of Small-Caliber Biodegradable Vascular Grafts in a Carotid Artery of the Sheep. *Pharmaceuticals* **2020**, *13*, 101. [CrossRef] [PubMed]
81. Chan, A.H.P.; Tan, R.P.; Michael, P.L.; Lee, B.S.L.; Vanags, L.Z.; Ng, M.K.C.; Bursill, C.A.; Wise, S.G. Evaluation of synthetic vascular grafts in a mouse carotid grafting model. *PLoS ONE* **2017**, *12*, e0174773. [CrossRef] [PubMed]
82. Mercado-Pagan, A.E.; Stahl, A.M.; Ramseier, M.L.; Behn, A.W.; Yang, Y. Synthesis and characterization of polycaprolactone urethane hollow fiber membranes as small diameter vascular grafts. *Mater. Sci. Eng. C Mater. Biol. Appl.* **2016**, *64*, 61–73. [CrossRef] [PubMed]
83. Liu, J.Y.; Swartz, D.D.; Peng, H.F.; Gugino, S.F.; Russell, J.A.; Andreadis, S.T. Functional tissue-engineered blood vessels from bone marrow progenitor cells. *Cardiovasc. Res.* **2007**, *75*, 618–628. [CrossRef]
84. Motlagh, D.; Allen, J.; Hoshi, R.; Yang, J.; Lui, K.; Ameer, G. Hemocompatibility evaluation of poly(diol citrate) in vitro for vascular tissue engineering. *J. Biomed. Mater. Res. Part A* **2007**, *82*, 907–916. [CrossRef] [PubMed]
85. Hashi, C.K.; Zhu, Y.; Yang, G.Y.; Young, W.L.; Hsiao, B.S.; Wang, K.; Chu, B.; Li, S. Antithrombogenic property of bone marrow mesenchymal stem cells in nanofibrous vascular grafts. *Proc. Natl. Acad. Sci. USA* **2007**, *104*, 11915–11920. [CrossRef]
86. Niklason, L.E.; Langer, R.S. Advances in tissue engineering of blood vessels and other tissues. *Transpl. Immunol.* **1997**, *5*, 303–306. [CrossRef]
87. Dahl, S.L.; Kypson, A.P.; Lawson, J.H.; Blum, J.L.; Strader, J.T.; Li, Y.; Manson, R.J.; Tente, W.E.; DiBernardo, L.; Hensley, M.T.; et al. Readily available tissue-engineered vascular grafts. *Sci. Transl. Med.* **2011**, *3*, 68ra9. [CrossRef] [PubMed]
88. Gui, L.; Niklason, L.E. Vascular Tissue Engineering: Building Perfusable Vasculature for Implantation. *Curr. Opin. Chem. Eng.* **2013**, *3*, 68–74. [CrossRef]
89. Habermehl, J.; Skopinska, J.; Boccafoschi, F.; Sionkowska, A.; Kaczmarek, H.; Laroche, G.; Mantovani, D. Preparation of ready-to-use, stockable and reconstituted collagen. *Macromol. Biosci.* **2005**, *5*, 821–828. [CrossRef]
90. Cen, L.; Liu, W.; Cui, L.; Zhang, W.; Cao, Y. Collagen Tissue Engineering: Development of Novel Biomaterials and Applications. *Pediatric Res.* **2008**, *63*, 492–496. [CrossRef] [PubMed]
91. Parenteau-Bareil, R.; Gauvin, R.; Berthod, F. Collagen-Based Biomaterials for Tissue Engineering Applications. *Materials* **2010**, *3*, 1863–1887. [CrossRef]
92. Dong, C.; Lv, Y. Application of Collagen Scaffold in Tissue Engineering: Recent Advances and New Perspectives. *Polymers* **2016**, *8*, 42. [CrossRef]
93. Long, T.; Yang, J.; Shi, S.S.; Guo, Y.P.; Ke, Q.F.; Zhu, Z.A. Fabrication of three-dimensional porous scaffold based on collagen fiber and bioglass for bone tissue engineering. *J. Biomed. Mater. Res. Part B Appl. Biomater.* **2015**, *103*, 1455–1464. [CrossRef]
94. Shoulders, M.D.; Raines, R.T. Collagen structure and stability. *Annu. Rev. Biochem.* **2009**, *78*, 929–958. [CrossRef]
95. Villa, M.M.; Wang, L.; Huang, J.; Rowe, D.W.; Wei, M. Bone tissue engineering with a collagen-hydroxyapatite scaffold and culture expanded bone marrow stromal cells. *J. Biomed. Mater. Res. Part B Appl. Biomater.* **2015**, *103*, 243–253. [CrossRef] [PubMed]
96. Wang, K.H.; Wan, R.; Chiu, L.H.; Tsai, Y.H.; Fang, C.L.; Bowley, J.F.; Chen, K.C.; Shih, H.N.; Lai, W.T. Effects of collagen matrix and bioreactor cultivation on cartilage regeneration of a full-thickness critical-size knee joint cartilage defects with subchondral bone damage in a rabbit model. *PLoS ONE* **2018**, *13*, e0196779. [CrossRef] [PubMed]
97. Panduranga Rao, K. Recent developments of collagen-based materials for medical applications and drug delivery systems. *J. Biomater. Sci. Polym. Ed.* **1996**, *7*, 623–645. [CrossRef] [PubMed]
98. Copes, F.; Pien, N.; Van Vlierberghe, S.; Boccafoschi, F.; Mantovani, D. Collagen-Based Tissue Engineering Strategies for Vascular Medicine. *Front. Bioeng. Biotechnol.* **2019**, *7*, 166. [CrossRef] [PubMed]
99. Konrad, P.; Dougan, P.; Bergqvist, D. Acute thrombogenicity of collagen coating of dacron grafts: An experimental study in sheep. *Eur. J. Vasc. Surg.* **1992**, *6*, 67–72. [CrossRef]

100. Udelsman, B.V.; Khosravi, R.; Miller, K.S.; Dean, E.W.; Bersi, M.R.; Rocco, K.; Yi, T.; Humphrey, J.D.; Breuer, C.K. Characterization of evolving biomechanical properties of tissue engineered vascular grafts in the arterial circulation. *J. Biomech.* **2014**, *47*, 2070–2079. [CrossRef]
101. Cai, Z.; Gu, Y.; Cheng, J.; Li, J.; Xu, Z.; Xing, Y.; Wang, C.; Wang, Z. Decellularization, cross-linking and heparin immobilization of porcine carotid arteries for tissue engineering vascular grafts. *Cell Tissue Bank* **2019**, *20*, 569–578. [CrossRef]
102. Gu, L.; Shan, T.; Ma, Y.-X.; Tay, F.R.; Niu, L. Novel Biomedical Applications of Crosslinked Collagen. *Trends Biotechnol.* **2019**, *37*, 464–491. [CrossRef]
103. Gough, J.E.; Scotchford, C.A.; Downes, S. Cytotoxicity of glutaraldehyde crosslinked collagen/poly(vinyl alcohol) films is by the mechanism of apoptosis. *J. Biomed. Mater. Res.* **2002**, *61*, 121–130. [CrossRef]
104. Additive Manufacturing of Vascular Grafts and Vascularized Tissue Constructs. *Tissue Eng. Part B Rev.* **2017**, *23*, 436–450. [CrossRef]
105. Brinkman, W.T.; Nagapudi, K.; Thomas, B.S.; Chaikof, E.L. Photo-Cross-Linking of Type I Collagen Gels in the Presence of Smooth Muscle Cells: Mechanical Properties, Cell Viability, and Function. *Biomacromolecules* **2003**, *4*, 890–895. [CrossRef]
106. Van Wachem, P.B.; Plantinga, J.A.; Wissink, M.J.B.; Beernink, R.; Poot, A.A.; Engbers, G.H.M.; Beugeling, T.; van Aken, W.G.; Feijen, J.; van Luyn, M.J.A. In vivo biocompatibility of carbodiimide-crosslinked collagen matrices: Effects of crosslink density, heparin immobilization, and bFGF loading. *J. Biomed. Mater. Res.* **2001**, *55*, 368–378. [CrossRef]
107. Alessandrino, A.; Chiarini, A.; Biagiotti, M.; Dal Prà, I.; Bassani, G.A.; Vincoli, V.; Settembrini, P.; Pierimarchi, P.; Freddi, G.; Armato, U. Three-Layered Silk Fibroin Tubular Scaffold for the Repair and Regeneration of Small Caliber Blood Vessels: From Design to in vivo Pilot Tests. *Front. Bioeng. Biotechnol.* **2019**, *7*, 356. [CrossRef] [PubMed]
108. Asakura, T.; Tanaka, T.; Tanaka, R. Advanced Silk Fibroin Biomaterials and Application to Small-Diameter Silk Vascular Grafts. *ACS Biomater. Sci. Eng.* **2019**, *5*, 5561–5577. [CrossRef]
109. Rockwood, D.N.; Preda, R.C.; Yücel, T.; Wang, X.; Lovett, M.L.; Kaplan, D.L. Materials fabrication from Bombyx mori silk fibroin. *Nat. Protoc.* **2011**, *6*, 1612–1631. [CrossRef] [PubMed]
110. Sericin Removal from Raw Bombyx mori Silk Scaffolds of High Hierarchical Order. *Tissue Eng. Part C Methods* **2014**, *20*, 431–439. [CrossRef] [PubMed]
111. Kunz, R.I.; Brancalhão, R.M.C.; Ribeiro, L.D.F.C.; Natali, M.R.M. Silkworm Sericin: Properties and Biomedical Applications. *BioMed Res. Int.* **2016**, *2016*, 8175701. [CrossRef]
112. Puerta, M.; Montoya, Y.; Bustamante, J.; Restrepo-Osorio, A. Potential Applications of Silk Fibroin as Vascular Implants: A Review. *Crit. Rev.™ Biomed. Eng.* **2019**, *47*, 365–378. [CrossRef]
113. Enomoto, S.; Sumi, M.; Kajimoto, K.; Nakazawa, Y.; Takahashi, R.; Takabayashi, C.; Asakura, T.; Sata, M. Long-term patency of small-diameter vascular graft made from fibroin, a silk-based biodegradable material. *J. Vasc. Surg.* **2010**, *51*, 155–164. [CrossRef]
114. Aper, T.; Teebken, O.E.; Steinhoff, G.; Haverich, A. Use of a Fibrin Preparation in the Engineering of a Vascular Graft Model. *Eur. J. Vasc. Endovasc. Surg.* **2004**, *28*, 296–302. [CrossRef]
115. Weisel, J.W.; Litvinov, R.I. Fibrin Formation, Structure and Properties. *Subcell. Biochem.* **2017**, *82*, 405–456.
116. Wolberg, A.S.; Campbell, R.A. Thrombin generation, fibrin clot formation and hemostasis. *Transfus. Apher. Sci.* **2008**, *38*, 15–23. [CrossRef]
117. Kim, J.; Ha, Y.; Kang, N.H. Effects of Growth Factors From Platelet-Rich Fibrin on the Bone Regeneration. *J. Craniofacial Surg.* **2017**, *28*, 860–865. [CrossRef] [PubMed]
118. Mallis, P.; Gontika, I.; Dimou, Z.; Panagouli, E.; Zoidakis, J.; Makridakis, M.; Vlahou, A.; Georgiou, E.; Gkioka, V.; Stavropoulos-Giokas, C.; et al. Short Term Results of Fibrin Gel Obtained from Cord Blood Units. A Preliminary in Vitro Study. *Bioengineering* **2019**, *6*, 66. [CrossRef] [PubMed]
119. Desai, C.B.; Mahindra, U.R.; Kini, Y.K.; Bakshi, M.K. Use of Platelet-Rich Fibrin over Skin Wounds: Modified Secondary Intention Healing. *J. Cutan. Aesthet. Surg.* **2013**, *6*, 35–37. [CrossRef] [PubMed]
120. Gelmetti, A.; Greppi, N.; Guez, S.; Grassi, F.; Rebulla, P.; Tadini, G. Cord blood platelet gel for the treatment of inherited epidermolysis bullosa. *Transfus. Apher. Sci.* **2018**, *57*, 370–373. [CrossRef]
121. Rebulla, P.; Pupella, S.; Santodirocco, M.; Greppi, N.; Villanova, I.; Buzzi, M.; De Fazio, N.; Grazzini, G. Multicentre standardisation of a clinical grade procedure for the preparation of allogeneic platelet concentrates from umbilical cord blood. *Blood Transfus.* **2016**, *14*, 73–79. [PubMed]

122. Singh, G.; Cordero, J.; Wiles, B.; Tembelis, M.N.; Liang, K.-L.; Rafailovich, M.; Simon, M.; Khan, S.U.; Bui, D.T.; Dagum, A.B. Development of In Vitro Bioengineered Vascular Grafts for Microsurgery and Vascular Surgery Applications. *Plast. Reconstr. Surg. Glob. Open* **2019**, *7*, e2264. [CrossRef]
123. Koch, S.; Flanagan, T.C.; Sachweh, J.S.; Tanios, F.; Schnoering, H.; Deichmann, T.; Ellä, V.; Kellomäki, M.; Gronloh, N.; Gries, T.; et al. Fibrin-polylactide-based tissue-engineered vascular graft in the arterial circulation. *Biomaterials* **2010**, *31*, 4731–4739. [CrossRef] [PubMed]
124. Koch, S.; Tschoeke, B.; Deichmann, T.; Ella, V.; Gronloh, N.; Gries, T.; Tolba, R.; Kellomäki, M.; Schmitz-Rode, T.; Jockenhoevel, S. Fibrin-based tissue engineered vascular graft in carotid artery position – the first in vivo experiences. *Thorac. Cardiovasc. Surg.* **2010**, *58*, MP25. [CrossRef]
125. Swartz, D.D.; Russell, J.A.; Andreadis, S.T. Engineering of fibrin-based functional and implantable small-diameter blood vessels. *Am. J. Physiol. Heart Circ. Physiol.* **2005**, *288*, H1451–H1460. [CrossRef]
126. Yang, L.; Li, X.; Wang, D.; Mu, S.; Lv, W.; Hao, Y.; Lu, X.; Zhang, G.; Nan, W.; Chen, H.; et al. Improved mechanical properties by modifying fibrin scaffold with PCL and its biocompatibility evaluation. *J. Biomater. Sci. Polym. Ed.* **2020**, *31*, 658–678. [CrossRef] [PubMed]
127. Wang, Y.; He, C.; Feng, Y.; Yang, Y.; Wei, Z.; Zhao, W.; Zhao, C. A chitosan modified asymmetric small-diameter vascular graft with anti-thrombotic and anti-bacterial functions for vascular tissue engineering. *J. Mater. Chem. B* **2020**, *8*, 568–577. [CrossRef] [PubMed]
128. Rinaudo, M. Chitin and chitosan: Properties and applications. *Prog. Polym. Sci.* **2006**, *31*, 603–632. [CrossRef]
129. Yao, Y.; Wang, J.; Cui, Y.; Xu, R.; Wang, Z.; Zhang, J.; Wang, K.; Li, Y.; Zhao, Q.; Kong, D. Effect of sustained heparin release from PCL/chitosan hybrid small-diameter vascular grafts on anti-thrombogenic property and endothelialization. *Acta Biomater.* **2014**, *10*, 2739–2749. [CrossRef]
130. Benhabiles, M.S.; Salah, R.; Lounici, H.; Drouiche, N.; Goosen, M.F.A.; Mameri, N. Antibacterial activity of chitin, chitosan and its oligomers prepared from shrimp shell waste. *Food Hydrocoll.* **2012**, *29*, 48–56. [CrossRef]
131. Huynh, T.N.; Tranquillo, R.T. Fusion of Concentrically Layered Tubular Tissue Constructs Increases Burst Strength. *Ann. Biomed. Eng.* **2010**, *38*, 2226–2236. [CrossRef]
132. Syedain, Z.H.; Graham, M.L. A completely biological "off-the-shelf" arteriovenous graft that recellularizes in baboons. *Sci. Transl. Med.* **2017**, *9*, eaan4209. [CrossRef]
133. Syedain, Z.; Reimer, J.; Lahti, M.; Berry, J.; Johnson, S.; Tranquillo, R.T. Tissue engineering of acellular vascular grafts capable of somatic growth in young lambs. *Nat. Commun.* **2016**, *7*, 12951. [CrossRef]
134. Cummings, C.L.; Gawlitta, D.; Nerem, R.M.; Stegemann, J.P. Properties of engineered vascular constructs made from collagen, fibrin, and collagen–fibrin mixtures. *Biomaterials* **2004**, *25*, 3699–3706. [CrossRef]
135. Arrigoni, C.; Chittò, A.; Mantero, S.; Remuzzi, A. Rotating versus perfusion bioreactor for the culture of engineered vascular constructs based on hyaluronic acid. *Biotechnol. Bioeng.* **2008**, *100*, 988–997. [CrossRef]
136. Lovett, M.; Eng, G.; Kluge, J.A.; Cannizzaro, C.; Vunjak-Novakovic, G.; Kaplan, D.L. Tubular silk scaffolds for small diameter vascular grafts. *Organogenesis* **2010**, *6*, 217–224. [CrossRef] [PubMed]
137. Li, X.; Xu, J.; Bartolák-Suki, E.; Jiang, J.; Tien, J. Evaluation of 1-mm-diameter endothelialized dense collagen tubes in vascular microsurgery. *J. Biomed. Mater. Res. Part B Appl. Biomater.* **2020**, *108*, 2441–2449. [CrossRef] [PubMed]
138. Zhang, L.; Ao, Q.; Wang, A.; Lu, G.; Kong, L.; Gong, Y.; Zhao, N.; Zhang, X. A sandwich tubular scaffold derived from chitosan for blood vessel tissue engineering. *J. Biomed. Mater. Res. Part A* **2006**, *77A*, 277–284. [CrossRef] [PubMed]
139. Skovrind, I.; Harvald, E.B.; Juul Belling, H.; Jørgensen, C.D.; Lindholt, J.S.; Andersen, D.C. Concise Review: Patency of Small-Diameter Tissue-Engineered Vascular Grafts: A Meta-Analysis of Preclinical Trials. *Stem Cells Transl. Med.* **2019**, *8*, 671–680. [CrossRef] [PubMed]
140. Wang, K.; Chen, X.; Pan, Y.; Cui, Y.; Zhou, X.; Kong, D.; Zhao, Q. Enhanced Vascularization in Hybrid PCL/Gelatin Fibrous Scaffolds with Sustained Release of VEGF. *BioMed Res. Int.* **2015**, *2015*, 865076. [CrossRef] [PubMed]
141. Kim, D.; Chung, J.J.; Jung, Y.; Kim, S.H. The effect of Substance P/Heparin conjugated PLCL polymer coating of bioinert ePTFE vascular grafts on the recruitment of both ECs and SMCs for accelerated regeneration. *Sci. Rep.* **2019**, *9*, 17083. [CrossRef]
142. Manske, M.; Bade, E.G. Growth Factor-Induced Cell Migration: Biology and Methods of Analysis. In *International Review of Cytology*; Jeon, K.W., Jarvik, J., Eds.; Academic Press: Cambridge, MA, USA, 1994; Volume 155, pp. 49–96.

143. Tillman, B.W.; Yazdani, S.K.; Lee, S.J.; Geary, R.L.; Atala, A.; Yoo, J.J. The in vivo stability of electrospun polycaprolactone-collagen scaffolds in vascular reconstruction. *Biomaterials* **2009**, *30*, 583–588. [CrossRef]
144. Wise, S.G.; Byrom, M.J.; Waterhouse, A.; Bannon, P.G.; Ng, M.K.C.; Weiss, A.S. A multilayered synthetic human elastin/polycaprolactone hybrid vascular graft with tailored mechanical properties. *Acta Biomater.* **2011**, *7*, 295–303. [CrossRef]
145. Li, Z.; Li, X.; Xu, T.; Zhang, L. Acellular Small-Diameter Tissue-Engineered Vascular Grafts. *Appl. Sci.* **2019**, *9*, 2864. [CrossRef]
146. Berglund, J.D.; Mohseni, M.M.; Nerem, R.M.; Sambanis, A. A biological hybrid model for collagen-based tissue engineered vascular constructs. *Biomaterials* **2003**, *24*, 1241–1254. [CrossRef]
147. Gong, W.; Lei, D.; Li, S.; Huang, P.; Qi, Q.; Sun, Y.; Zhang, Y.; Wang, Z.; You, Z.; Ye, X.; et al. Hybrid small-diameter vascular grafts: Anti-expansion effect of electrospun poly ε-caprolactone on heparin-coated decellularized matrices. *Biomaterials* **2016**, *76*, 359–370. [CrossRef] [PubMed]
148. Thomas, L.V.; Nair, P.D. Influence of Mechanical Stimulation in the Development of a Medial Equivalent Tissue-Engineered Vascular Construct using a Gelatin-g-Vinyl Acetate Co-Polymer Scaffold. *J. Biomater. Sci. Polym. Ed.* **2012**, *23*, 2069–2087. [CrossRef] [PubMed]
149. Mun, C.H.; Jung, Y.; Kim, S.-H.; Kim, H.C.; Kim, S.H. Effects of Pulsatile Bioreactor Culture on Vascular Smooth Muscle Cells Seeded on Electrospun Poly (lactide-co-ε-caprolactone) Scaffold. *Artif. Organs* **2013**, *37*, E168–E178. [CrossRef]
150. Jirofti, N.; Mohebbi-Kalhori, D.; Samimi, A.; Hadjizadeh, A.; Kazemzadeh, G.H. Fabrication and characterization of a novel compliant small-diameter PET/PU/PCL triad-hybrid vascular graft. *Biomed. Mater.* **2020**, *15*, 055004. [CrossRef]
151. Khodadoust, M.; Mohebbi-Kalhori, D.; Jirofti, N. Fabrication and Characterization of Electrospun Bi-Hybrid PU/PET Scaffolds for Small-Diameter Vascular Grafts Applications. *Cardiovasc. Eng. Technol.* **2018**, *9*, 73–83. [CrossRef] [PubMed]
152. Nguyen, T.H.; Padalhin, A.R.; Seo, H.S.; Lee, B.T. A hybrid electrospun PU/PCL scaffold satisfied the requirements of blood vessel prosthesis in terms of mechanical properties, pore size, and biocompatibility. *J. Biomater. Sci. Polym. Ed.* **2013**, *24*, 1692–1706. [CrossRef] [PubMed]
153. Lu, G.; Cui, S.J.; Geng, X.; Ye, L.; Chen, B.; Feng, Z.G.; Zhang, J.; Li, Z.Z. Design and preparation of polyurethane-collagen/heparin-conjugated polycaprolactone double-layer bionic small-diameter vascular graft and its preliminary animal tests. *Chin. Med. J.* **2013**, *126*, 1310–1316.
154. Gilbert, T.W.; Sellaro, T.L.; Badylak, S.F. Decellularization of tissues and organs. *Biomaterials* **2006**, *27*, 3675–3683. [CrossRef]
155. Gilpin, A.; Yang, Y. Decellularization Strategies for Regenerative Medicine: From Processing Techniques to Applications. *BioMed Res. Int.* **2017**, *2017*, 9831534. [CrossRef]
156. Crapo, P.M.; Gilbert, T.W.; Badylak, S.F. An overview of tissue and whole organ decellularization processes. *Biomaterials* **2011**, *32*, 3233–3243. [CrossRef]
157. Chen, S.-G.; Ugwu, F.; Li, W.-C.; Caplice, N.M.; Petcu, E.; Yip, S.P.; Huang, C.-L. Vascular Tissue Engineering: Advanced Techniques and Gene Editing in Stem Cells for Graft Generation. *Tissue Eng. Part B Rev.* **2020**. [CrossRef] [PubMed]
158. Huai, G.; Qi, P.; Yang, H.; Wang, Y. Characteristics of α-Gal epitope, anti-Gal antibody, α1,3 galactosyltransferase and its clinical exploitation (Review). *Int. J. Mol. Med.* **2016**, *37*, 11–20. [CrossRef]
159. Galili, U. α1,3Galactosyltransferase knockout pigs produce the natural anti-Gal antibody and simulate the evolutionary appearance of this antibody in primates. *Xenotransplantation* **2013**, *20*, 267–276. [CrossRef]
160. Galili, U. Significance of the evolutionary α1,3-galactosyltransferase (GGTA1) gene inactivation in preventing extinction of apes and old world monkeys. *J. Mol. Evol.* **2015**, *80*, 1–9. [CrossRef] [PubMed]
161. Wu, L.-C.; Kuo, Y.-J.; Sun, F.-W.; Chen, C.-H.; Chiang, C.-J.; Weng, P.-W.; Tsuang, Y.-H.; Huang, Y.-Y. Optimized decellularization protocol including α-Gal epitope reduction for fabrication of an acellular porcine annulus fibrosus scaffold. *Cell Tissue Bank* **2017**, *18*, 383–396. [CrossRef] [PubMed]
162. Macher, B.A.; Galili, U. The Galalpha1,3Galbeta1,4GlcNAc-R (alpha-Gal) epitope: A carbohydrate of unique evolution and clinical relevance. *Biochim. Biophys. Acta* **2008**, *1780*, 75–88. [CrossRef] [PubMed]
163. Yang, H.; Wu, Z. Genome Editing of Pigs for Agriculture and Biomedicine. *Front. Genet.* **2018**, *9*, 360. [CrossRef]
164. Available online: https://www.organdonor.gov/ (accessed on 25 October 2020).

165. Kim, D.H.; Sohn, S.K.; Kim, J.G.; Suh, J.S.; Lee, K.S.; Lee, K.B. Clinical impact of hyperacute graft-versus-host disease on results of allogeneic stem cell transplantation. *Bone Marrow Transplant.* **2004**, *33*, 1025–1030. [CrossRef]
166. Chinen, J.; Buckley, R.H. Transplantation immunology: Solid organ and bone marrow. *J. Allergy Clin. Immunol.* **2010**, *125* (Suppl. 2), S324–S335. [CrossRef]
167. Keane, T.J.; Badylak, S.F. Biomaterials for tissue engineering applications. *Semin. Pediatric Surg.* **2014**, *23*, 112–118. [CrossRef]
168. Gilbert, T.W.; Freund, J.M.; Badylak, S.F. Quantification of DNA in biologic scaffold materials. *J. Surg. Res.* **2009**, *152*, 135–139. [CrossRef] [PubMed]
169. Zhou, S.; Wang, Y.; Zhang, K.; Cao, N.; Yang, R.; Huang, J.; Zhao, W.; Rahman, M.; Liao, H.; Fu, Q. The Fabrication and Evaluation of a Potential Biomaterial Produced with Stem Cell Sheet Technology for Future Regenerative Medicine. *Stem Cells Int.* **2020**, *2020*, 9567362. [CrossRef] [PubMed]
170. Gerli, M.F.M.; Guyette, J.P.; Evangelista-Leite, D.; Ghoshhajra, B.B.; Ott, H.C. Perfusion decellularization of a human limb: A novel platform for composite tissue engineering and reconstructive surgery. *PLoS ONE* **2018**, *13*, e0191497. [CrossRef]
171. Balestrini, J.L.; Gard, A.L.; Liu, A.; Leiby, K.L.; Schwan, J.; Kunkemoeller, B.; Calle, E.A.; Sivarapatna, A.; Lin, T.; Dimitrievska, S.; et al. Production of decellularized porcine lung scaffolds for use in tissue engineering. *Integr. Biol.* **2015**, *7*, 1598–1610. [CrossRef]
172. Mallis, P.; Katsimpoulas, M.; Kostakis, A.; Dipresa, D.; Korossis, S.; Papapanagiotou, A.; Kassi, E.; Stavropoulos-Giokas, C.; Michalopoulos, E. Vitrified Human Umbilical Arteries as Potential Grafts for Vascular Tissue Engineering. *Tissue Eng. Regen. Med.* **2020**, *17*, 285–299. [CrossRef]
173. Bakbak, S.; Kayacan, R.; Akkuş, O. Effect of collagen fiber orientation on mechanical properties of cortical bone. *J. Biomech.* **2011**, *44*, 11. [CrossRef]
174. Sokolis, D.P. Passive mechanical properties and structure of the aorta: Segmental analysis. *Acta Physiol.* **2007**, *190*, 277–289. [CrossRef]
175. Sokolis, D.P. Passive mechanical properties and constitutive modeling of blood vessels in relation to microstructure. *Med. Biol. Eng. Comput.* **2008**, *46*, 1187–1199. [CrossRef]
176. Rosenberg, N.; Martinez, A.; Sawyer, P.N.; Wesolowski, S.A.; Postlethwait, R.W.; Dillon, M.L., Jr. Tanned collagen arterial prosthesis of bovine carotid origin in man. Preliminary studies of enzyme-treated heterografts. *Ann. Surg.* **1966**, *164*, 247–256. [CrossRef] [PubMed]
177. Guler, S.; Aydin, H.M.; Lü, L.-X.; Yang, Y. Improvement of Decellularization Efficiency of Porcine Aorta Using Dimethyl Sulfoxide as a Penetration Enhancer. *Artif. Organs* **2018**, *42*, 219–230. [CrossRef] [PubMed]
178. Williams, C.; Liao, J.; Joyce, E.M.; Wang, B.; Leach, J.B.; Sacks, M.S.; Wong, J.Y. Altered structural and mechanical properties in decellularized rabbit carotid arteries. *Acta Biomater.* **2009**, *5*, 993–1005. [CrossRef] [PubMed]
179. Kajbafzadeh, A.-M.; Khorramirouz, R.; Kameli, S.M.; Hashemi, J.; Bagheri, A. Decellularization of Human Internal Mammary Artery: Biomechanical Properties and Histopathological Evaluation. *Biores. Open Access* **2017**, *6*, 74–84. [CrossRef] [PubMed]
180. Lin, C.H.; Hsia, K.; Tsai, C.H.; Ma, H.; Lu, J.H.; Tsay, R.Y. Decellularized porcine coronary artery with adipose stem cells for vascular tissue engineering. *Biomed. Mater.* **2019**, *14*, 045014. [CrossRef]
181. Singh, C.; Wong, C.S.; Wang, X. Medical Textiles as Vascular Implants and Their Success to Mimic Natural Arteries. *J. Funct. Biomater.* **2015**, *6*, 500. [CrossRef]
182. Pennel, T.; Fercana, G.; Bezuidenhout, D.; Simionescu, A.; Chuang, T.-H.; Zilla, P.; Simionescu, D. The performance of cross-linked acellular arterial scaffolds as vascular grafts; pre-clinical testing in direct and isolation loop circulatory models. *Biomaterials* **2014**, *35*, 6311–6322. [CrossRef] [PubMed]
183. Zhao, P.; Li, X.; Fang, Q.; Wang, F.; Ao, Q.; Wang, X.; Tian, X.; Tong, H.; Bai, S.; Fan, J. Surface modification of small intestine submucosa in tissue engineering. *Regen. Biomater.* **2020**, *7*, 339–348. [CrossRef] [PubMed]
184. Parmaksiz, M.; Elçin, A.E.; Elçin, Y.M. Decellularization of Bovine Small Intestinal Submucosa. *Methods Mol. Biol.* **2018**, *1577*, 129–138. [PubMed]
185. Hussein, K.H.; Park, K.M.; Lee, Y.S.; Woo, J.S.; Kang, B.J.; Choi, K.Y.; Kang, K.S.; Woo, H.M. New insights into the pros and cons of cross-linking decellularized bioartificial organs. *Int. J. Artif. Organs* **2017**, *40*, 136–141. [CrossRef]

186. Daugs, A.; Hutzler, B.; Meinke, M.; Schmitz, C.; Lehmann, N.; Markhoff, A.; Bloch, O. Detergent-Based Decellularization of Bovine Carotid Arteries for Vascular Tissue Engineering. *Ann. Biomed. Eng.* **2017**, *45*, 2683–2692. [CrossRef]
187. Mancuso, L.; Gualerzi, A.; Boschetti, F.; Loy, F.; Cao, G. Decellularized ovine arteries as small-diameter vascular grafts. *Biomed. Mater.* **2014**, *9*, 045011. [CrossRef]
188. Sandusky, G.E.; Lantz, G.C.; Badylak, S.F. Healing comparison of small intestine submucosa and ePTFE grafts in the canine carotid artery. *J. Surg. Res.* **1995**, *58*, 415–420. [CrossRef] [PubMed]
189. Chemla, E.S.; Morsy, M. Randomized clinical trial comparing decellularized bovine ureter with expanded polytetrafluoroethylene for vascular access. *Br. J. Surg.* **2009**, *96*, 34–39. [CrossRef] [PubMed]
190. Katzman, H.E.; Glickman, M.H.; Schild, A.F.; Fujitani, R.M.; Lawson, J.H. Multicenter evaluation of the bovine mesenteric vein bioprostheses for hemodialysis access in patients with an earlier failed prosthetic graft. *J. Am. Coll. Surg.* **2005**, *201*, 223–230. [CrossRef]
191. Cho, S.W.; Lim, S.H.; Kim, I.K.; Hong, Y.S.; Kim, S.S.; Yoo, K.J.; Park, H.Y.; Jang, Y.; Chang, B.C.; Choi, C.Y.; et al. Small-diameter blood vessels engineered with bone marrow-derived cells. *Ann. Surg.* **2005**, *241*, 506–515. [CrossRef]
192. Porzionato, A.; Stocco, E.; Barbon, S.; Grandi, F.; Macchi, V.; De Caro, R. Tissue-Engineered Grafts from Human Decellularized Extracellular Matrices: A Systematic Review and Future Perspectives. *Int. J. Mol. Sci.* **2018**, *19*, 4117. [CrossRef]
193. Development and Characterization of Acellular Allogeneic Arterial Matrices. *Tissue Eng. Part A* **2012**, *18*, 471–483. [CrossRef] [PubMed]
194. Teebken, O.E.; Puschmann, C.; Rohde, B.; Burgwitz, K.; Winkler, M.; Pichlmaier, A.M.; Weidemann, J.; Haverich, A. Human iliac vein replacement with a tissue-engineered graft. *VASA* **2009**, *38*, 60–65. [CrossRef]
195. Olausson, M.; Patil, P.B.; Kuna, V.K.; Chougule, P.; Hernandez, N.; Methe, K.; Kullberg-Lindh, C.; Borg, H.; Ejnell, H.; Sumitran-Holgersson, S. Transplantation of an allogeneic vein bioengineered with autologous stem cells: A proof-of-concept study. *Lancet* **2012**, *380*, 230–237. [CrossRef]
196. Rodríguez-Rodríguez, V.E.; Martínez-González, B.; Quiroga-Garza, A.; Reyes-Hernández, C.G.; de la Fuente-Villarreal, D.; de la Garza-Castro, O.; Guzmán-López, S.; Elizondo-Omaña, R.E. Human Umbilical Vessels: Choosing the Optimal Decellularization Method. *ASAIO J.* **2018**, *64*, 575–580. [CrossRef]
197. Velarde, F.; Castañeda, V.; Morales, E.; Ortega, M.; Ocaña, E.; Álvarez-Barreto, J.; Grunauer, M.; Eguiguren, L.; Caicedo, A. Use of Human Umbilical Cord and Its Byproducts in Tissue Regeneration. *Front. Bioeng. Biotechnol.* **2020**, *8*, 117. [CrossRef]
198. Asmussen, I.; Kjeldsen, K. Intimal ultrastructure of human umbilical arteries. Observations on arteries from newborn children of smoking and nonsmoking mothers. *Circ. Res.* **1975**, *36*, 579–589. [CrossRef] [PubMed]
199. Longo, L.D.; Reynolds, L.P. Some historical aspects of understanding placental development, structure and function. *Int. J. Dev. Biol.* **2010**, *54*, 237–255. [CrossRef] [PubMed]
200. Oblath, R.W.; Buckley, F.O., Jr.; Donnelly, W.A.; Green, R.M.; Deweese, J.A. Human umbilical veins and autogenous veins as canine arterial bypass grafts. *Ann. Surg.* **1978**, *188*, 158–161. [CrossRef] [PubMed]
201. Andersen, L.I.; Nielsen, O.M.; Buchardt Hansen, H.J. Umbilical vein bypass in patients with severe lower limb ischemia: A report of 121 consecutive cases. *Surgery* **1985**, *97*, 294–299. [PubMed]
202. Sato, O.; Okamoto, H.; Takagi, A.; Miyata, T.; Takayama, Y. Biodegradation of glutaraldehyde-tanned human umbilical vein grafts. *Surg. Today* **1995**, *25*, 901–905. [CrossRef] [PubMed]
203. Klinkert, P.; Post, P.N.; Breslau, P.J.; van Bockel, J.H. Saphenous vein versus PTFE for above-knee femoropopliteal bypass. A review of the literature. *Eur. J. Vasc. Endovasc. Surg.* **2004**, *27*, 357–362. [CrossRef]
204. Aalders, G.J.; van Vroonhoven, T.J.M.V. Polytetrafluoroethylene versus human umbilical vein in above-knee femoropopliteal bypass: Six-year results of a randomized clinical trial. *J. Vasc. Surg.* **1992**, *16*, 816–824. [CrossRef]
205. Neufang, A.; Espinola-Klein, C.; Dorweiler, B.; Messow, C.M.; Schmiedt, W.; Vahl, C.F. Femoropopliteal prosthetic bypass with glutaraldehyde stabilized human umbilical vein (HUV). *J. Vasc. Surg.* **2007**, *46*, 280–288. [CrossRef]
206. Kerdjoudj, H.; Berthelemy, N.; Rinckenbach, S.; Kearney-Schwartz, A.; Montagne, K.; Schaaf, P.; Lacolley, P.; Stoltz, J.F.; Voegel, J.C.; Menu, P. Small vessel replacement by human umbilical arteries with polyelectrolyte film-treated arteries: In vivo behavior. *J. Am. Coll. Cardiol.* **2008**, *52*, 1589–1597. [CrossRef]

207. Kerdjoudj, H.; Boura, C.; Marchal, L.; Dumas, D.; Schaff, P.; Voegel, J.C.; Stoltz, J.F.; Menu, P. Decellularized umbilical artery treated with thin polyelectrolyte multilayer films: Potential use in vascular engineering. *Bio-Med. Mater. Eng.* **2006**, *16* (Suppl. 4), S123–S129.
208. Gui, L.; Muto, A.; Chan, S.A.; Breuer, C.K.; Niklason, L.E. Development of decellularized human umbilical arteries as small-diameter vascular grafts. *Tissue Eng. Part A* **2009**, *15*, 2665–2676. [CrossRef] [PubMed]
209. Mallis, P.; Gontika, I.; Poulogiannopoulos, T.; Zoidakis, J.; Vlahou, A.; Michalopoulos, E.; Chatzistamatiou, T.; Papassavas, A.; Stavropoulos-Giokas, C. Evaluation of decellularization in umbilical cord artery. *Transplant. Proc.* **2014**, *46*, 3232–3239. [CrossRef] [PubMed]
210. Tuan-Mu, H.Y.; Chang, Y.H.; Hu, J.J. Removal of an abluminal lining improves decellularization of human umbilical arteries. *Sci. Rep.* **2020**, *10*, 10556. [CrossRef] [PubMed]
211. Chakhunashvili, K.; Kiladze, M.G.; Chakhunashvili, D.; Karalashvili, L.; Kakabadze, Z. A three-dimensional scaffold from decellularized human umbilical artery for bile duct reconstruction. *Ann. Ital. Chir.* **2019**, *90*, 165–173. [PubMed]
212. Mallis, P.; Sokolis, D.P.; Makridakis, M.; Zoidakis, J. Insights into Biomechanical and Proteomic Characteristics of Small Diameter Vascular Grafts Utilizing the Human Umbilical Artery. *Biomedicines* **2020**, *8*, 280. [CrossRef]
213. Madden, R.L.; Lipkowitz, G.S.; Browne, B.J.; Kurbanov, A. A comparison of cryopreserved vein allografts and prosthetic grafts for hemodialysis access. *Ann. Vasc. Surg.* **2005**, *19*, 686–691. [CrossRef]
214. Jarrett, F.; Mahood, B.A. Long-term results of femoropopliteal bypass with stabilized human umbilical vein. *Am. J. Surg.* **1994**, *168*, 111–114. [CrossRef]
215. Hoenicka, M.; Schrammel, S.; Bursa, J.; Huber, G.; Bronger, H.; Schmid, C.; Birnbaum, D.E. Development of endothelium-denuded human umbilical veins as living scaffolds for tissue-engineered small-calibre vascular grafts. *J. Tissue Eng. Regen. Med.* **2013**, *7*, 324–336. [CrossRef]
216. Katsimpoulas, M.; Morticelli, L.; Gontika, I.; Kouvaka, A.; Mallis, P.; Dipresa, D.; Böer, U.; Soudah, B.; Haverich, A.; Michalopoulos, E.; et al. Biocompatibility and immunogenecity of decellularized allogeneic aorta in the orthotopic rat model. *Tissue Eng. Part A.* **2019**, *25*, 399–415. [CrossRef]
217. Nuyttens, B.P.; Thijs, T.; Deckmyn, H.; Broos, K. Platelet adhesion to collagen. *Thromb. Res.* **2011**, *127*, S26–S29. [CrossRef]
218. Kumar, R.A.; Dong, J.-F.; Thaggard, J.A.; Cruz, M.A.; López, J.A.; McIntire, L.V. Kinetics of GPIbalpha-vWF-A1 tether bond under flow: Effect of GPIbalpha mutations on the association and dissociation rates. *Biophys. J.* **2003**, *85*, 4099–4109. [CrossRef]
219. Pugh, N.; Simpson, A.M.; Smethurst, P.A.; de Groot, P.G.; Raynal, N.; Farndale, R.W. Synergism between platelet collagen receptors defined using receptor-specific collagen-mimetic peptide substrata in flowing blood. *Blood* **2010**, *115*, 5069–5079. [CrossRef] [PubMed]
220. Zhou, M.; Liu, Z.; Liu, C.; Jiang, X.; Wei, Z.; Qiao, W.; Ran, F.; Wang, W.; Qiao, T.; Liu, C. Tissue engineering of small-diameter vascular grafts by endothelial progenitor cells seeding heparin-coated decellularized scaffolds. *J. Biomed. Mater. Res. Part B Appl. Biomater.* **2012**, *100*, 111–120. [CrossRef] [PubMed]
221. Kaushal, S.; Amiel, G.E.; Guleserian, K.J.; Shapira, O.M.; Perry, T.; Sutherland, F.W.; Rabkin, E.; Moran, A.M.; Schoen, F.J.; Atala, A.; et al. Functional small-diameter neovessels created using endothelial progenitor cells expanded ex vivo. *Nat. Med.* **2001**, *7*, 1035–1040. [CrossRef] [PubMed]
222. Ma, X.; He, Z.; Li, L.; Liu, G.; Li, Q.; Yang, D.; Zhang, Y.; Li, N. Development and in vivo validation of tissue-engineered, small-diameter vascular grafts from decellularized aortae of fetal pigs and canine vascular endothelial cells. *J. Cardiothorac. Surg.* **2017**, *12*, 101. [CrossRef]
223. Row, S.; Peng, H.; Schlaich, E.M.; Koenigsknecht, C.; Andreadis, S.T.; Swartz, D.D. Arterial grafts exhibiting unprecedented cellular infiltration and remodeling in vivo: The role of cells in the vascular wall. *Biomaterials* **2015**, *50*, 115–126. [CrossRef]
224. Peck, M.; Dusserre, N.; McAllister, T.N.; L'Heureux, N. Tissue engineering by self-assembly. *Mater. Today* **2011**, *14*, 218–224. [CrossRef]
225. Jun, I.; Han, H.-S.; Edwards, J.R.; Jeon, H. Electrospun Fibrous Scaffolds for Tissue Engineering: Viewpoints on Architecture and Fabrication. *Int. J. Mol. Sci.* **2018**, *19*, 745. [CrossRef]
226. Papaioannou, T.G.; Manolesou, D.; Dimakakos, E.; Tsoucalas, G.; Vavuranakis, M.; Tousoulis, D. 3D Bioprinting Methods and Techniques: Applications on Artificial Blood Vessel Fabrication. *Acta Cardiol. Sin.* **2019**, *35*, 284–289.

227. Vacanti, J.P.; Langer, R. Tissue engineering: The design and fabrication of living replacement devices for surgical reconstruction and transplantation. *Lancet* **1999**, *354* (Suppl. 1), Si32–Si34. [CrossRef]
228. L'Heureux, N.; Dusserre, N.; Konig, G.; Victor, B.; Keire, P.; Wight, T.N.; Chronos, N.A.; Kyles, A.E.; Gregory, C.R.; Hoyt, G.; et al. Human tissue-engineered blood vessels for adult arterial revascularization. *Nat. Med.* **2006**, *12*, 361–365. [CrossRef] [PubMed]
229. L'Heureux, N.; Pâquet, S.; Labbé, R.; Germain, L.; Auger, F.A. A completely biological tissue-engineered human blood vessel. *FASEB J.* **1998**, *12*, 47–56.
230. McAllister, T.N.; Maruszewski, M.; Garrido, S.A.; Wystrychowski, W.; Dusserre, N.; Marini, A.; Zagalski, K.; Fiorillo, A.; Avila, H.; Manglano, X.; et al. Effectiveness of haemodialysis access with an autologous tissue-engineered vascular graft: A multicentre cohort study. *Lancet* **2009**, *373*, 1440–1446. [CrossRef]
231. Niu, H.; Zhou, H.; Wang, H. Electrospinning: An Advanced Nanofiber Production Technology. In *Energy Harvesting Properties of Electrospun Nanofibers*; IOP Publishing: Bristol, UK, 2019; pp. 1-1–1-44.
232. Mirjalili, M.; Zohoori, S. Review for application of electrospinning and electrospun nanofibers technology in textile industry. *J. NanoStruct. Chem.* **2016**, *6*, 207–213. [CrossRef]
233. Li, Z.; Wang, C. Effects of Working Parameters on Electrospinning. In *One-Dimensional Nanostructures: Electrospinning Technique and Unique Nanofibers*; Li, Z., Wang, C., Eds.; Springer: Berlin/Heidelberg, Germany, 2013; pp. 15–28.
234. Hasan, A.; Memic, A.; Annabi, N.; Hossain, M.; Paul, A.; Dokmeci, M.R.; Dehghani, F.; Khademhosseini, A. Electrospun scaffolds for tissue engineering of vascular grafts. *Acta Biomater.* **2014**, *10*, 11–25. [CrossRef] [PubMed]
235. Davidenko, N.; Schuster, C.F.; Bax, D.V.; Farndale, R.W.; Hamaia, S.; Best, S.M.; Cameron, R.E. Evaluation of cell binding to collagen and gelatin: A study of the effect of 2D and 3D architecture and surface chemistry. *J. Mater. Sci. Mater. Med.* **2016**, *27*, 148. [CrossRef]
236. Soletti, L.; Nieponice, A.; Hong, Y.; Ye, S.H.; Stankus, J.J.; Wagner, W.R.; Vorp, D.A. In vivo performance of a phospholipid-coated bioerodable elastomeric graft for small-diameter vascular applications. *J. Biomed. Mater. Res. Part A* **2011**, *96*, 436–448. [CrossRef]
237. Ju, Y.M.; Ahn, H.; Arenas-Herrera, J.; Kim, C.; Abolbashari, M.; Atala, A.; Yoo, J.J.; Lee, S.J. Electrospun vascular scaffold for cellularized small diameter blood vessels: A preclinical large animal study. *Acta Biomater.* **2017**, *59*, 58–67. [CrossRef]
238. Du, F.; Wang, H.; Zhao, W.; Li, D.; Kong, D.; Yang, J.; Zhang, Y. Gradient nanofibrous chitosan/poly ε-caprolactone scaffolds as extracellular microenvironments for vascular tissue engineering. *Biomaterials* **2012**, *33*, 762–770. [CrossRef]
239. Gu, B.K.; Choi, D.J.; Park, S.J.; Kim, M.S.; Kang, C.M.; Kim, C.-H. 3-dimensional bioprinting for tissue engineering applications. *Biomater. Res.* **2016**, *20*, 12. [CrossRef]
240. Tamay, D.G.; Dursun Usal, T.; Alagoz, A.S.; Yucel, D.; Hasirci, N.; Hasirci, V. 3D and 4D Printing of Polymers for Tissue Engineering Applications. *Front. Bioeng. Biotechnol.* **2019**, *7*, 164. [CrossRef] [PubMed]
241. Abaci, A.; Guvendiren, M. Designing Decellularized Extracellular Matrix-Based Bioinks for 3D Bioprinting. *Adv. Healthc. Mater.* **2020**, e2000734. [CrossRef] [PubMed]
242. Jang, J.; Park, H.-J.; Kim, S.-W.; Kim, H.; Park, J.Y.; Na, S.J.; Kim, H.J.; Park, M.N.; Choi, S.H.; Park, S.H.; et al. 3D printed complex tissue construct using stem cell-laden decellularized extracellular matrix bioinks for cardiac repair. *Biomaterials* **2017**, *112*, 264–274. [CrossRef] [PubMed]
243. Ligon, S.C.; Liska, R.; Stampfl, J.; Gurr, M.; Mülhaupt, R. Polymers for 3D Printing and Customized Additive Manufacturing. *Chem. Rev.* **2017**, *117*, 10212–10290. [CrossRef] [PubMed]
244. Mosadegh, B.; Xiong, G.; Dunham, S.; Min, J.K. Current progress in 3D printing for cardiovascular tissue engineering. *Biomed. Mater.* **2015**, *10*, 034002. [CrossRef]
245. Freeman, S.; Ramos, R.; Alexis Chando, P.; Zhou, L.; Reeser, K.; Jin, S.; Soman, P.; Ye, K. A bioink blend for rotary 3D bioprinting tissue engineered small-diameter vascular constructs. *Acta Biomater.* **2019**, *95*, 152–164. [CrossRef]
246. Jia, W.; Gungor-Ozkerim, P.S.; Zhang, Y.S.; Yue, K.; Zhu, K.; Liu, W.; Pi, Q.; Byambaa, B.; Dokmeci, M.R.; Shin, S.R.; et al. Direct 3D bioprinting of perfusable vascular constructs using a blend bioink. *Biomaterials* **2016**, *106*, 58–68. [CrossRef]
247. Gao, B.; Yang, Q.; Zhao, X.; Jin, G.; Ma, Y.; Xu, F. 4D Bioprinting for Biomedical Applications. *Trends Biotechnol.* **2016**, *34*, 746–756. [CrossRef]

248. Rastogi, P.; Kandasubramanian, B. Breakthrough in the printing tactics for stimuli-responsive materials: 4D printing. *Chem. Eng. J.* **2019**, *366*, 264–304. [CrossRef]
249. Castro, N.J.; Meinert, C.; Levett, P.; Hutmacher, D.W. Current developments in multifunctional smart materials for 3D/4D bioprinting. *Curr. Opin. Biomed. Eng.* **2017**, *2*, 67–75. [CrossRef]
250. Suntornnond, R.; An, J.; Chua, C.K. Bioprinting of Thermoresponsive Hydrogels for Next Generation Tissue Engineering: A Review. *Macromol. Mater. Eng.* **2017**, *302*, 1600266. [CrossRef]
251. De Souza Ferreira, S.B.; Moço, T.D.; Borghi-Pangoni, F.B.; Junqueira, M.V.; Bruschi, M.L. Rheological, mucoadhesive and textural properties of thermoresponsive polymer blends for biomedical applications. *J. Mech. Behav. Biomed. Mater.* **2016**, *55*, 164–178. [CrossRef] [PubMed]
252. Reyes-Ortega, F. 3-pH-responsive polymers: Properties, synthesis and applications. In *Smart Polymers and their Applications*; Aguilar, M.R., San Román, J., Eds.; Woodhead Publishing: Southston, UK, 2014; pp. 45–92.
253. Ratemi, E. 5-pH-responsive polymers for drug delivery applications. In *Stimuli Responsive Polymeric Nanocarriers for Drug Delivery Applications*; Makhlouf, A.S.H., Abu-Thabit, N.Y., Eds.; Woodhead Publishing: Southston, UK, 2018; Volume 1, pp. 121–141.
254. Adedoyin, A.A.; Ekenseair, A.K. Biomedical applications of magneto-responsive scaffolds. *Nano Res.* **2018**, *11*, 5049–5064. [CrossRef]
255. Lv, C.; Sun, X.-C.; Xia, H.; Yu, Y.-H.; Wang, G.; Cao, X.-W.; Li, S.-X.; Wang, Y.-S.; Chen, Q.-D.; Yu, Y.-D.; et al. Humidity-responsive actuation of programmable hydrogel microstructures based on 3D printing. *Sens. Actuators B Chem.* **2018**, *259*, 736–744. [CrossRef]
256. Bobis, S.; Jarocha, D.; Majka, M. Mesenchymal stem cells: Characteristics and clinical applications. *Folia Histochem. Cytobiol.* **2006**, *44*, 215–230. [PubMed]
257. Gimble, J.M.; Bunnell, B.A.; Chiu, E.S.; Guilak, F. Concise review: Adipose-derived stromal vascular fraction cells and stem cells: Let's not get lost in translation. *Stem Cells* **2011**, *29*, 749–754. [CrossRef]
258. Dominici, M.; Le Blanc, K.; Mueller, I.; Slaper-Cortenbach, I.; Marini, F.C.; Krause, D.S.; Deans, R.J.; Keating, A.; Prockop, D.J.; Horwitz, E.M. Minimal criteria for defining multipotent mesenchymal stromal cells. The International Society for Cellular Therapy position statement. *Cytotherapy* **2006**, *8*, 315–317. [CrossRef]
259. Viswanathan, S.; Shi, Y.; Galipeau, J.; Krampera, M.; Leblanc, K.; Martin, I.; Nolta, J.; Phinney, D.G.; Sensebe, L. Mesenchymal stem versus stromal cells: International Society for Cell & Gene Therapy (ISCT®;) Mesenchymal Stromal Cell committee position statement on nomenclature. *Cytotherapy* **2019**, *21*, 1019–1024.
260. Xiao, X.; Li, N.; Zhang, D.; Yang, B.; Guo, H.; Li, Y. Generation of Induced Pluripotent Stem Cells with Substitutes for Yamanaka's Four Transcription Factors. *Cellular Reprogram.* **2016**, *18*, 281–297. [CrossRef]
261. Peng, G.-Y.; Lin, Y.; Li, J.-J.; Wang, Y.; Huang, H.-Y.; Shen, Z.-Y. The Application of Induced Pluripotent Stem Cells in Pathogenesis Study and Gene Therapy for Vascular Disorders: Current Progress and Future Challenges. *Stem Cells Int.* **2019**, *2019*, 9613258. [CrossRef]
262. Wiegand, C.; Banerjee, I. Recent advances in the applications of iPSC technology. *Curr. Opin. Biotechnol.* **2019**, *60*, 250–258. [CrossRef] [PubMed]
263. Zacharias, D.G.; Nelson, T.J.; Mueller, P.S.; Hook, C.C. The science and ethics of induced pluripotency: What will become of embryonic stem cells? *Mayo Clin. Proc.* **2011**, *86*, 634–640. [CrossRef] [PubMed]
264. Mendicino, M.; Fan, Y.; Griffin, D.; Gunter, K.C.; Nichols, K. Current state of U.S. Food and Drug Administration regulation for cellular and gene therapy products: Potential cures on the horizon. *Cytotherapy* **2019**, *21*, 699–724. [CrossRef]
265. Badylak, S.F.; Gilbert, T.W. Immune response to biologic scaffold materials. *Semin. Immunol.* **2008**, *20*, 109–116. [CrossRef] [PubMed]
266. Elliott, M.B.; Ginn, B.; Fukunishi, T.; Bedja, D.; Suresh, A.; Chen, T.; Inoue, T.; Dietz, H.C.; Santhanam, L.; Mao, H.-Q.; et al. Regenerative and durable small-diameter graft as an arterial conduit. *Proc. Natl. Acad. Sci. USA* **2019**, *116*, 12710–12719. [CrossRef]

Publisher's Note: MDPI stays neutral with regard to jurisdictional claims in published maps and institutional affiliations.

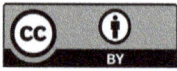

© 2020 by the authors. Licensee MDPI, Basel, Switzerland. This article is an open access article distributed under the terms and conditions of the Creative Commons Attribution (CC BY) license (http://creativecommons.org/licenses/by/4.0/).

MDPI
St. Alban-Anlage 66
4052 Basel
Switzerland
Tel. +41 61 683 77 34
Fax +41 61 302 89 18
www.mdpi.com

Bioengineering Editorial Office
E-mail: bioengineering@mdpi.com
www.mdpi.com/journal/bioengineering

www.ingramcontent.com/pod-product-compliance
Lightning Source LLC
LaVergne TN
LVHW070547100526
838202LV00012B/410